ADVANCE PRAISE FOR
JONNY BOWDEN'S SHAPE UP!

"Now everyone can have Jonny Bowden in their corner. . . . His *Shape Up!* is a must-read and should be in everybody's library."

—Richard N. Firshein, D.O.,
author of *The Nutraceutical Revolution*

"With wit and clarity, Bowden challenges nutritional myth after nutritional myth, all the while emphasizing that when it comes to staying fit, the key is to understand your individual needs."

—Robert Epstein, Ph.D., editor, *Psychology Today*

"Jonny Bowden is one of those ultra-rare fitness trainers who understands real nutrition. This unique book combines both his motivational and nutritional strengths. All of us could do well to adopt the *Shape Up!* eating plan."

—Allan Spreen, M.D., author of *Nutritionally Incorrect*

"Writing with clarity and force, Jonny Bowden provides authoritative and enthusiastic guidance on weight and health management. Highly recommended!"

—Jeffrey R. Wilbert, Ph.D., clinical psychologist and
author of *Fattitudes: Beat Self-Defeat and Win Your War with Weight.*

"At last a 'diet' program that doctors can recommend to their patients. State-of the-art nutritional advice you won't hear from everyone else, coupled with an action plan that produces results."

—David Leonardi, M.D.,
medical director, Cenegenics Medical Institute

"Jonny Bowden makes losing weight and being healthy as easy as A-B-C. His *Shape Up!* will help you make good nutrition a part of your life."

—Harvey Diamond, author of *Fit for Life*

"Jonny Bowden is a highly knowledgeable educator whose expertise and direction have provided results for hundreds of people over the years. His instincts seem to always be right."

—Jon Giswold, author *Basic Training*

"Jonny Bowden is one of the brightest minds in the field of nutrition today. This book is one of the few that incorporates all of the latest nutrition research, and in a way that can help you achieve your health goals."

—Robert Crayhon, M.S.,
author of *Nutrition Made Simple* and *The Carnitine Miracle*

"You will not want to put this book down. You want to keep reading because you just know that Jonny Bowden has *the* answer."

—Linda Lizotte, R.D., C.D.N.

"Jonny Bowden is brilliant. In a very thoughtful manner, he offers the keys to weight control. *Shape Up!* is a clever, smart, and fun way to lose weight, increase your energy, get fit, and learn to love to eat again. Enjoy it!"

—Oz Garcia, author of *The Balance*

"In my fifteen years as a trainer and a coach in the fitness industry I have prided myself and my company on our ability to get results, particularly with actors and models whose careers depend on achieving them. Jonathan Bowden has been my teacher; his input has been the 'secret ingredient' for many of my greatest successes."

—Bill Humphries, chairman, LightChaser Sports

JONNY BOWDEN'S SHAPE UP!

JONNY

The Eight-Week Plan to

BOWDEN'S

Transform Your Body,

SHAPE UP!

Your Health and Your Life

JONNY BOWDEN

PERSEUS PUBLISHING

Cambridge, Massachusetts

Perseus Publishing is a member of the Perseus Books Group
Cover design by Steve Cooley
Text design by Jeffrey P. Williams
Illustrations by Meryl Henderson
Set in 11-point Minion by Perseus Publishing Services
First printing, March 2001

Visit us on the World Wide Web at http://www.perseusbooks.com

Perseus Books are available at special discounts for bulk purchases in the U.S. by corporations, institutions, and other organizations. For more information, please contact the Special Markets Department at HarperCollins Publishers, 10 East 53rd Street, New York, NY 10022, or call 1–212–207–7528.

To my beloved partner, lover,
best friend and inspiration,

Cassandra Creech

The cake* under which all the rest is icing

*organic of course

Information doesn't change anyone.
Inspiration does.

—Bernie Siegal, M.D.
Love, Medicine, and Miracles

CONTENTS

ACKNOWLEDGMENTS

I've been amazingly fortunate to have on my speed-dial a veritable brain trust in nutrition, medicine and research whose collective intellectual wattage could easily power the Star Wars system with some left to spare. When you've got this bunch at your disposal, it becomes a lot easier to take on the medical and nutritional establishment. I may be David going up against Goliath, but having the input of this group makes me feel like my slingshot is backed up with an Uzi.

So with enormous gratitude I acknowledge my mentors in nutrition and health whom I am inordinately proud to call colleagues:

C. Leigh Broadhurst, Ph.D.
Barry Sears, Ph.D.
Ann Louise Gittleman, M.S., C.N.S.
Dave Leonardi, M.D.
Allan Spreen, M.D.
Linda Lizotte, R.D.
    and especially. . .
Robert Crayhon, Ph.D.

Acknowledgments and kudos to the entire staff of the Designs for Health Institute, who are slowly but surely accomplishing their honorable mission of bringing nutrition education into the twenty-first century and with whom I am proud to be associated.

To the God of Education for giving me some of the best teachers in the world, among them Scott Frasier for psychology at the New School for Social Research, Rob Kapilow for music and Dr. Ernest van den Haag for everything else.

Equinox Fitness Clubs, which had the good sense and trust to hire me as a de facto "intellectual-at-large" and where I was let loose to hone my craft and hopefully help them hone theirs.

Oz Garcia, who started me on the path.

i-Village, which gave me a forum, constant support, a staff like Allison Rand and Emily Lapkin, and an audience of some of the most wonderful women in the world.

www.eYada.com for giving me the best job in the world.

And especially to my friend Liz Neporent, with whom I agree about virtually nothing, but without whom I would not have a career.

Sharon Kolberg, the Wordsmith Queen, for her magical eye, invaluable skill and gifted ability to tweak.

William Goldman, whom I never met, but from whom I learned most of what I know about great nonfiction writing.

Linda Konner for her superhuman patience and her invaluable assistance in putting together the proposal and placing it in the perfect hands of the perfect editor, Marnie Cochran.

My mother, from whom I learned unconditional love.

My father, from whom I learned compassion and wisdom.

My brother, Jeffrey Bowden, and my sister-in-law, Dr. Nancy Fiedler, for forcing me to learn the habit of being able to back-up everything I say.

My niece, Cadence, and my nephew, Pace, just because they think I'm cool even though they care nothing about what I write.

And most especially Werner Erhard, wherever you are. If you only knew. (Come to think of it, I'm sure you do.)

And of course Cassandra because I love her so much she deserves to be mentioned twice.

MORE
ACKNOWLEDGMENTS

Because so much of Shape Up is about integrating the whole person, about being healthy in addition to just being lean, about being how you are in the world—which is so much more than just a number on the scale—and because so much of my personal philosophy about health is based on connections with other people, with community, with something larger than myself . . . I want to acknowledge the enormous contribution to my soul of people who have sustained me through the years with their friendship and presence in my life, and without whom I would not be who I am. Therefore, without these people I would not have written this book: Billy Stritch, Scott Ellis, Peter Breger, Mike Mandel, Bill Humphries, Lauree Dash, Jackie Balough, Randy Graff, Susan Wood, Adrian Zmed, Jeanine Tsori, Danny Troob, Kathryn Grody, Liz Neporent, Oz Garcia, and especially Oliver and Jennifer Becaud, who honored my wife and me with their friendship and trust when they made us godparents of their beautiful daughter Leslie.

WHAT IS THE SHAPE UP PROGRAM?

> The good physician treats the disease,
> but the great physician treats the patient.
>
> —SIR WILLIAM OSLER

I once gave a seminar in which I asked, "How many of you in the audience would like to lose five pounds or more and get in a little bit better shape?" Virtually the whole audience raised their hands. Then I said, "How many of you feel you know exactly what you need to do to make that happen?" Again, a sea of hands, though maybe fewer than before. Finally: "And how many of you who *know* what you *should* be doing are actually *doing* it?"

Lots of nervous giggles, fewer hands this time around.

My work with hundreds of clients during ten years of personal training and nutrition consulting has taught me one thing time and time again: that giving "pure information" on how to lose weight *never works*. For too long the diet industry and the diet "dictocrats" have looked at the *subject* of weight loss rather than at the *person having to lose the weight*. A perfect program that doesn't take into account the *person doing the program* is like an exquisitely made Armani dress in the wrong size. If the tailor doesn't take into account the client's measurements, the finest fabrics in the world won't look good on her body. A weight loss program that doesn't take into account individual factors like commitment, self-esteem, sexual confidence, impulse control, goal setting, addictions, behavior patterns, body image and social support, not to mention the background issues of metabolic type, genetics, ethnic heritage and hormones, is virtually doomed to failure.

This program is about making that off-the-rack dress fit perfectly.

And that's why the Shape Up program is fundamentally different from any you've done before.

For years, we've heard that diets don't work. We've heard that up to 95 percent of the people who lose weight on diets gain it back again.

ception is reality, and the perception is this: Diets equal failure, deprivation and misery.

Actually, the truth is a little more shaded.

It's not that diets don't work. It's that diet *programs* don't work.

The problem isn't in the food plans themselves, which often are quite
good, assuming you're lucky enough to choose one that is a good fit with
your individual metabolic biochemistry. The problem is more basic:
People don't like being told what to do.

Now the conventional wisdom says otherwise. Virtually every publish-
er of diet books knows it to be a "fact" that people want to be told *exactly*
what they can and can't eat, they want a plan, and they want it simple,
clear and easy to follow. And in the short run, that's probably true. There's
a great comfort and relief in giving up control to the authority of an
expert who will guide you down a specific path, who promises that if you
just stick to the letter of the law you will get the results you want, with a
minimum of effort and pain. An attractive proposition, and it's the reason
that diet books sell. The formula is tried and true: Design a program that
tells people exactly what they can and cannot do, and promise them that
if they follow the plan *exactly* as specified they will lose weight.

Except that they don't follow it.

And it's not just diets. There are dozens of published studies showing
that people don't follow prescribed regimens for asthma, depression,
chronic illness, diabetes, kidney disease and just about any other condition you care to name. (One study showed that 59 out of 100 glaucoma
patients failed to use the prescribed eyedrops as directed even though
doing so would significantly reduce their chances of going blind!)
Everyone "knows" they should exercise, but 80 percent of Americans
don't, and only a small minority of those who do exercise follow a rigorous prescribed program. The conclusion is inescapable: *It's hard to follow
a program that someone else imposes on you, even when you think it's good
for you.* The problem with a diet isn't the diet. The problem with a "diet"
is following a structured program of someone else's design that eventually feels to you like imposed deprivation and self-denial.

Think for a moment of any activity in your life that you or someone
close to you really likes to do. My nephew, Pace, is a great example. This
twelve-year-old is a natural athlete and takes to skateboarding like a fox to
chickens. He doesn't need an externally imposed regimen to go outside
and get on the board. In fact, you need to practically duct tape him inside
the house to get him to keep away from it. And for most people, that's just
the way it is. No one has to "make" a golf fanatic go to the course every

Sunday, and no one has to "make" an avid reader pick up a book, and no one has to "make" an avid shopper go to the mall.

This may seem like a simple point, but it really is the core of why diet programs fail and why the Shape Up program is different. *People don't fail when they design their own lives according to what they want to do.* The trick is getting clear on what we want our lives to be like and then choosing strategies that get us there. Think about it: Doesn't that sound a lot different than the usual concept of a diet? I promised you earlier that you won't have to go on a diet during this program, at least not in any traditional sense of the word. Here's why: If you go on any diet at all during this program, it will be one that *you* make up. It will be one of your own design. We're going to build a house together here, you and I, but you're going to be the architect and I'm going to be the contractor. I'll be here to give you all kinds of advice about what materials are best to use for the kind of house *you* want to build, what strategies are most likely to work for the kind of goals *you* want to achieve, and what tools are most likely to be effective for the kind of construction work that *you* choose to do, but make no mistake, the final design will be yours, and you will own it.

So with that in mind, let's talk a little more about this hateful concept of "dieting."

Suppose we weren't talking about food but instead about money. Suppose you kept maxing out your credit cards, were constantly in debt, didn't know where your money was disappearing to and were always fighting to keep your head above water financially. Sound familiar? Now it would be sheer lunacy to expect that if you continued exactly on the same path, your money problems would suddenly, miraculously disappear. If what you were doing was working so well, you wouldn't be in debt, right?

So you go to a financial consultant who analyzes your income, your spending patterns, your expectations and the like. Logically, you'd expect the advisor to give you some suggestions for change. Some of those changes might be really easy; some might be difficult. Some changes might require that you give up certain purchases, that you cut back on others, that you even work within a budget for a while until you master the skills required for financial solvency and make them into habits.

Ultimately, though, the way you spend your money needs to be *your* choice. Only *you* can decide your priorities, what's worth saving for, and what's worth spending on. And these decisions are going to be, by definition, based entirely on your individual circumstances. Maybe you've always wanted a yacht but the amount of financial sacrifice you'd have to make to own one is just not worth it. But maybe for someone else it *would* be worth it. A third person might not even like boats and would be happy just to have the mortgage paid and enough money for an occasional vacation. A fourth person might decide that having the yacht wouldn't really require much of a financial sacrifice at all—she might just have to choose between the yacht and a private jet. The financial advisor can only give you a menu of options; he can help you assess your personal situation and lay out strategies to help you reach your goals. But he can't tell you what those goals should be.

Well, why should it be any different with food and fitness?

I can't tell you what your goal should be. But if you tell me what it is—and if it's healthy and it makes sense—I can tell you how to get there.

In that context, let's revisit the term "diet." "Diet" doesn't have to be a dirty word. Right now, it connotes magic pills, quick fixes, starvation, deprivation and obsession. Let's throw all that out and redefine it as something else.

A plan for action. Of your own making.

A diet is simply a *program of change in the areas of behavior and attitudes about food and exercise*. In the original Greek, "diet" meant "a manner of living." A diet is just a way of putting some kind of limits on a style of eating that is for some reason not producing the desired results. What those limits are, how they are constructed, and what they exclude and include are going to be decisions *you* are going to make during this program. And you're not going to make them from a position of fear and anxiety; you're going to make them from a position of power and strength.

You can make some easy changes right now, this minute, and you will be on the path to changing your life. That's what this program is about.

How far you want to go on that path is up to you.

See, there really are two very different questions here, and it's important to understand the difference. One is "*How* do I lose weight?" The other is "*Should* I do it in the first place?" You can't really begin to answer the first till you've given some thought to the second.

Which is the question that everyone skips over.

I can't tell you whether losing weight is a good idea for you, or if it'll make your life better, or if it's worth the work. I can tell you *how* to do it if you *choose* to do it, or at least I can share with you strategies that have worked for many people in the past. But I cannot tell you that this is a journey you ought to be taking. The only person who can answer that one for you is reading this book right now.

Look, let's pretend we're in the gold rush, circa 1850. Everyone is coming to town looking to strike it rich in the hills. You come in, prospector's pan in hand, and you ask me, a longtime resident of the town, which is the best route to take to find the gold.

I can tell you that the folks who have been going south have been coming home really disappointed. I can tell you that the word on the street is that if you go north, you'll find a lot of fool's gold and that while it's a pretty scenic route, no one's coming back rich. And I can tell you that the folks who have chosen to go west are coming back with smiles on their faces and seem to be pretty friendly with the local banker.

What I *can't* do is this: I can't tell you if it's worth the climb. I can't tell you whether getting rich is a worthwhile goal, or whether money will ultimately make you happy, or if you would be better off pursuing something else.

And in the same way, I cannot tell you that you "should" lose weight. I cannot tell anyone whether it's worth it or not, especially since exactly what each person's going to have to do to achieve it will be quite different in every single case. What I *can* do is help you successfully navigate the path, once you choose to take it. How rocky or how smooth that particular path is going to be depends on a zillion factors that we can't fully anticipate, and whether you want to stay on it will be something only you can decide. My goal is to help you do two things: be successful on whatever path you choose to take and feel good about whatever path you choose.

To begin the journey, you're not going to have to learn complicated formulas or percentages, you're not going to be told you have to cut out any specific food or food group and you're not going to have to count calories, fat grams, carb grams or any other kind of grams. I'll give you some options for using those strategies later on *should you choose to*, but it'll be in a very different context than you're used to, and in any case, you definitely don't "have to."

You're also not going to have to do an exercise program that Linda Hamilton would have found tough while preparing for *Terminator II*.

In fact, when it comes right down to it, you're not going to "have" to do anything at all.

Now if that's making you nervous, please stay with me. Because right about now, you're probably asking, "Well, if this isn't a conventional diet, and it isn't a set of hard and fast rules, how is it going to *work*? This weight won't come off by itself—it never has. What *do* I have to do? How's it going to happen?"

Good questions, and there are very good answers.

Here's what *will* happen. You will learn a lot about how you put on weight and why. (Some of the reasons may surprise you.) And you'll learn, maybe for the first time in a form you can use, how to do something about it in a way that works for *you*.

I can almost hear you saying, "But I already *know* why I have put this weight on that I can't get rid of. It's because I — (fill in the blank: eat too much food, eat too much fat, don't have any discipline, can't get motivated, don't work out, etc.).

Well, maybe.

But if you're already so sure that the reason you got fatter than you want to be is whatever you filled in the blank with, how come you bought this book? If you already know the reason you're getting wet is that you forgot to open your umbrella, why not just open the damn umbrella and be done with it?

Maybe because it's not as simple as that.

This program is about weight loss, but more important, it's about *your* weight loss, which, please believe me, is going to be significantly different from your friend's weight loss, or your cousin's weight loss, or some Hollywood star's weight loss. (In fact, even if you *are* a Hollywood star, it's going to be different from some *other* Hollywood star's). It's about us designing a program together that fits *your* measurements, *your* temperament, and *your* lifestyle and that takes into account the zillions of factors that make you completely metabolically and biochemically unique.

This program is about making that off-the-rack dress we spoke about earlier fit.

You will learn a lot about your body chemistry, how your body makes and releases fat, how it creates cravings that seem to defeat your best attempts to "tough it out," how it betrays you by refusing to change despite dozens of failed attempts to trick it into losing weight. You're also going to learn, in a way you can absolutely understand and appreciate, why most of the dietary and weight loss information you've been getting is not only dead wrong but actually works *against* your best efforts to change your body. But this won't be some idle intellectual exercise. You'll also learn how you can harness that knowledge to empower you rather than enslave you. You'll learn how your body and mind work together when it comes to weight loss, and how virtually impossible it is to deal with one without the other. In the process of doing so, you'll also probably discover why most weight loss programs fail miserably and why this one won't.

A pretty outrageous statement. You're probably thinking right now, "How do you *know* that? How can you *possibly* say I won't fail on this program?"

And the answer is . . .

. . . because you can't. If there are no "rules" to break, there is no way to fail. I know you picked up this book for one reason and one reason only, which was to find a way to finally change your body and feel better about yourself, so I don't want to go too far afield here, but I will let you in on a little secret: This book is about giving you choices. And about making you a more powerful person.

We're going to use that power to change both your weight and how you feel about it, but make no mistake—that power, once applied, has a way of taking on a life of its own. Master your weight, master your life. Once the power to do that is out of the box, there's no putting it back in.

This book is about you taking charge of your life and being the author of your own destiny. When you control what happens in your life, you control your weight. As you follow this program and stay with this book, I guarantee you will come out as a more powerful person than you were when you started. What you do with this power is up to you. One thing you cannot do is give it back. So even if you choose not to use it to lose weight right now—I'm sure you *will*, but let's just say for some reason you choose not to—you will always have it and be able to enlist it at any time in your life. Like a pair of magical infrared glasses that let you see through things, it will always be available to you to pick up and try anytime you really want to understand what's really going on with you and your body. When you're ready to do something about it, you will know exactly *what* to do. Not because I'm going to tell you, not because I'm going to give you a set of unbendable rules to follow, not because *my* diet information is better than the *last* diet book you read, but because the Shape Up program is about *you* discovering what put *your* weight on in the first place, what *keeps* it on and what *you* need to do to taket it off.

So what's the bad news?

Well, you're going to have to do some of the work. You'll have help along the way of course—but if you're expecting to find a program that spells out for you exactly what to eat with the precise portions all neatly laid out for you, I'm afraid you've come to the wrong book. But you know what? If you've read even this far, you know deep down *those programs don't work anyway*. If they did, you wouldn't be *Jonny Bowden's Shape-Up!* You'd simply pick up one of the dozens of women's magazines that have new ten-day programs in every issue and you'd follow one of them. Maybe you've already done that. In fact, maybe you've done it more times than you care to think about. And maybe, just maybe, that's why you're reading this book.

If it is, then you've come to the right place. Whether you know it yet or not, you've probably realized that the only real way to change your body is to learn about *your* body—not your neighbor's, not your husband's, not someone you work with who found some great diet that worked for her, but *your* body.

This program is going to show you how small changes that can easily be incorporated into your life can wind up making a big difference in your health, your weight and your state of mind. (It's also going to show you how to make *bigger* changes, if and when you decide you want to.) It's not a program that's going to demand you give up huge chunks of time, eat in a completely different way, join a gym or completely change your life. You can do all those things, of course, but you don't *have* to in order to get the benefits of the program.

Fitness, health and wellness are not all-or-nothing propositions. Sure, most people—as they begin to drop weight, feel better and have more energy—find that they want to do more, take the next step and get deeper into this new life-enhancing way of being. Some become fanatics (well, there are worse things you could become fanatical about). Some become athletes. (Take Pam, for example. A schoolteacher from Colorado, she hadn't exercised regularly since college. With two kids and a busy schedule teaching school, she felt that she had "let herself go" in the decade since graduating. About a year after doing my program she wrote to tell me that she had just completed her first mini-triathlon.) Some so love the way they feel and the sense of empowerment that goes with it that they want to spread the word to others and have even gone on to become personal trainers and coaches themselves! If that turns out to be you, great. More than one fitness and nutrition guru started his professional life by becoming his own best client (for example, *me*).

But you don't have to become any of those things—a fanatic, a marathoner or a personal trainer—to lose weight and benefit from this program. All you really have to do—and I promise you I won't be using that expression very much anymore—is keep an open mind and be willing to do the homework assignments you'll find throughout the book.

So if you've never gotten your feet wet before—or if you've been out of the pond for a while—this is the place to start. You're going to take concrete, measurable, meaningful steps, one at a time, that will lead to a healthier, fitter, leaner you. You don't have to be a committed marathoner to get the benefits of jogging, and you don't have to follow a rigorous diet and exercise program with religious fervor to lose weight. You don't have to devote your life to fitness to benefit from this program. And you don't need to be a fanatic to get healthier; you just need to be willing to throw out some of your old assumptions about what healthy eating looks like.

The take home point here is this: Health and weight loss and self-esteem are impossible to separate from one another. And all three are close cousins of empowerment. It's very hard to "just" take weight off, especially if weight has been a long-standing problem for you. It's impossible to do it successfully and not learn something profound about yourself in the process. Some of these things are concrete and physical—like how certain foods affect you, your moods, your energy, your skin, your cravings. Some are psychological and spiritual—like about keeping your word (to yourself and others), being able to follow through and learning how to work through a problem or an obstacle. The point is this: Start with weight loss and it will automatically impact other areas of your life.

Consider the following: Every time you try to stop doing something destructive—whether it's smoking, eating junk food or even participating in a destructive relationship at work or at home—and you don't actually *do* it, something happens. You stop believing in your own word. You stop believing in your own power. You feel in some way diminished. So it stands to reason that whenever you begin to actually *do* what you say you're going to do, you feel empowered. And that's what this program is about.

As the old saying goes, "If you *keep doing* what you *say you're going to do*, and what you *say* is going to happen *keeps happening*. . .

after a while. . .

. . . your word becomes law in the universe."

When you've completed the Shape Up program, you'll not only like the way the person in the mirror looks, you'll understand her a lot better.

DIETING OR STRATEGY?

The Completely Unique Laboratory: You

Nutrition is for real people.
Statistical human beings hold no interest.

—ROGER WILLIAMS, PH.D.,
BIOCHEMICAL INDIVIDUALITY

Stop for a minute and do this exercise: Picture the busiest, most crowded, active street in a downtown location in New York City. Got it? Now think about *every single thing* that could be happening simultaneously within the confines of that city block. Think about *every single piece of information* you could amass about anything and everything and everybody within the limits of that city block. (If you really want to get the point of this, go make a list, and when you run out of things to list, return to this page.)

Back already? OK, what did *you* think of?

Here are some things you might have noticed on that imaginary street. And maybe some things you didn't.

If you look at this block just from the point of view of a local utilities company, you're going to see the thousands of electrical connections supplying apartments, offices, buildings, and the myriad of underground cables and wiring complexes. If you're a phone company person, you might survey the zillions of connections, switching boxes, and interconnections that service the corded and wireless and satellite communications networks all going on at any given time. If you're a real estate person, you might look at the condition (and value) of the many buildings on the block and notice the different states of repair or disrepair that they're in. Which ones need renovation, and which ones are spanking new? How about the elevators? Do some need inspection? What else did you notice? Maybe there's a drug deal or some illegal gambling going on down the street. How many cops are patrolling the street? Maybe some of the trucks stuck in traffic are putting some heavy emissions into the air. What is that cute, interesting couple intensely engaged in deep conversation talking about? What deals are being closed in the high towers of that office building over there? What relationships are being formed? What relationships are *ending*? How's business for that fruit stand on the corner?

It should be immediately apparent that if you took all the combined information on everything that was happening on that busy block at any given point in time, you could easily fill a book the size of the yellow pages. And it should *also* be pretty obvious that you could write a similar-sized *but different* book based on the information on any street in America (or in the world). Even though the streets might have things in common—people, buildings, electrical cables, phone lines, automobiles, water mains, deal making, relationships—none of the books written about them would be identical.

I want you to play with me for one more moment. Suppose now that a large city planning firm came to your town and tried to sell you on a plan for how to renovate the block *you personally* live on. But it was the same plan they had used for every other block, in every other city, in every other country. No matter that there was no illegal activity on your block; you got the same number of cops as the roughest part of town. You have two broken gas mains? Doesn't matter; you get the same attention to your gas mains as the block up the street that has all new equipment. Just got all new traffic lights installed? You still get the same budget for traffic lights as the block in the next town that has a broken light on every corner.

What do you think of this plan?

Ah, you're beginning to get the picture.

Look, when it comes to complexity and function and uniqueness, your body is *just like a city block*. And just as different and special and unique as any city block in the world. While you have many organs and functions and physiological characteristics and psychological traits in common with virtually every other human on the planet, the particular way they arrange and compile and function, with their particular needs and quirks and tastes and peculiarities and strengths and weaknesses and signaling mechanisms, is unalterably, uniquely you and different from *any other person on the planet*. Yet orthodox medicine and traditional dietetics have continued to try to sell you the same old one-size-fits-all renovation plan for your body as if that yellow pages–sized book of your personal information were exactly the same as everyone else's.

Let's go back to our mythical city planning company with its one-size-fits-all renovation plan. Once in a while, just by the law of averages, a plan like that happens to land on a street whose needs match it perfectly, and there is a successful "renovation." When that happens, all the people who were lucky enough to live on that street rejoice and sing the praises of the planning company, and people all across the country want to hire that same planning company to have *their* streets renovated with the exact same plan.

In the diet world *the same thing happens*. Once in a while, by luck or good grace, someone happens to connect with a one-size-fits-all plan that just *happens* to be their size, like grabbing an off-the-rack suit that just happens to fit perfectly. It *can* happen. And if it happens to enough people, which it *will do* just by the law of averages, you invariably get a new diet book, a new diet guru, a new "system" that everyone swears by until, invariably, the plan is applied to enough people on whom it doesn't work and it eventually falls out of favor.

When it comes to diet and weight loss, orthodox medicine has been operating in this way for years—just change plans as often as the popular media.

Look, we all have voice boxes, fingers, noses, eyes, ears and skin. In that way we're completely alike. Yet if that were all that mattered, how is it you can pick up the phone and call any friend of yours with whom you talk frequently and just say hi and they'll know instantly who's on the other end? Why are our fingerprints different? Why does one person's skin tan easily and tolerate hours on the beach while another's blisters at the first exposure to the sun?

The answer is this: biochemical individuality. And you have a far greater chance of success on a weight loss program if you completely understand this all-important principle, so let's take some time to really understand what it's about.

Biochemical individuality. In the simplest sense, it means that we are all unique. The term itself was first coined by the brilliant researcher (and discoverer of pantothenic acid) Dr. Roger Williams, who wrote a book by the same name. Dr. Williams's seminal book chronicles in great detail the amazing variations in both form and function that are most often hidden beneath the skin.

Here's a tiny sampling: From the *Atlas of Human Anatomy*, he reproduces illustrations of nineteen different laboratory specimen human stomachs of dramatically different shape and size and does the same for seventeen different livers. He reports on differences—*dramatic* differences—among *normal healthy infants* in leukocytes, neutrophils, eosinophils, basophils, lymphocytes and monocytes. He reports on huge differences in the musculature of the *pectoralis minor* muscle and on the variations in the amount of islet tissue in the pancreas. He suggests that the potential rate of production for *insulin alone* probably varies throughout a ten-fold or greater range, and that the number of insulin-producing cells in the pancreas varies from 200,000 to 2.5 million. This, by the way, in *normal* people. The thyroid gland in normal people varies from a weight of 8 grams to 50 grams. Pepsin, a digestive enzyme produced by the stomach and one of the two most important functional constituents of gastric juice, varies in the *normal stomach* by a *thousand-fold*. Testicular weight in normal males can range from 2 to 10 grams (the visual for this produces an interesting reaction if you're doing a lecture presentation).

"The particular insertion of a muscle in the back of a hand can make the difference between a concert pianist and a person who's all thumbs," stated Dr. Alexander Ballin, in a lecture about biochemical individuality and vitamin needs. Twenty-two percent of people have differences in the structure of this muscle; 13 percent don't have the muscle at all; 1 percent have *two* muscles.

I'll spare you the rigorous, dry scientific terminology of Dr. Williams's book and the countless others that have come after it and sum it all up for you in two words: *Everybody's different*. That's why the Shape Up plan doesn't offer you a specific diet but rather suggests a specific *menu* of possibilities. That doesn't mean there aren't good guidelines, just that there isn't a one-size-fits-all absolute. The same dietary strategy will not work for everyone, and the sooner we *really* understand that, deep down in the bone marrow of our souls, the better off we'll be.

Sometimes a person will read something that I've written about picking a strategy and will get very distressed because she'll think I said that she's going to have to give up a favorite food (something I almost never say, by the way). She'll write in or call in and ask, quite agitated, "*You mean I can't eat wheat?*" I usually answer, "I don't know, *can* you? Let's find out." The fact is, you can eat whatever you want, but what you eat, how much and how frequently are all decisions that only you can make. Every dietary action you take is a decision. Actions have consequences, but if there's one thing the work of Dr. Roger Williams and his colleagues has taught us, it's this: *Those consequences are going to be different for different people.* Genetics, metabolic type, metabolic efficiency, age, sex, enzyme activity, blood type and who knows what else all form a particular metabolic stew that results in a unique package as distinct as your DNA.

My friend and colleague Dr. Dave Leonardi is married to a lovely woman named Lisa, who remains aerobically slim and flat-bellied even after two babies. One night over dinner, I asked him the secret of Lisa's remarkable ability to maintain her figure well into her late thirties and through two pregnancies. "A combination of things," he said. "But the main one is that she picked the right parents!" He told me that he had taken glucometer (blood sugar) readings on her after she ate a candy bar, and found that her blood sugar barely moved—it behaved in the same way as *his* did when he ate a portion of broccoli! Broccoli and candy have very different effects on blood sugar, but even within these parameters we have to respect that there are huge individual variations in response. While Lisa still has to work out and eat right, the fact is that she is genetically blessed with a carbohydrate metabolism that is a lot more forgiving than most, which makes it a lot easier to maintain low body fat. Dr. Dave, on the other hand, has to work a lot harder to get the same results, and his metabolism is a lot less forgiving of dietary transgressions. Not fair? Sure ain't. But that's just how it is.

Louis Pasteur was the author of the "germ theory" of disease. He believed that by learning the nature and behavior of different bacteria and viruses, you could learn what illness was about. For decades he labored to do just that, but toward the end of his life he had a change of heart, or, more accurately, an expansion of vision. On his deathbed he was rumored to have said four words: "Look to the host."

The actions of bacteria and viruses are important for the infectious disease specialist to know, but it's also important to know that they *do not behave in exactly the same way in every single person*. If they did, everyone who was exposed to a virus or a cold would get that cold or virus. This just isn't the case. (Ever notice that when a cold goes around your office, some people get a mild case of it, while others are out for two weeks and still others don't get it at all?) A hurricane is a hurricane, but its effect on different houses along the seashore is quite different—it will blow the roof off some of them while others are left relatively unscathed.

And so it is with food. And with everything else in life.

The lesson from this is as simple and pure and ancient as wisdom itself: Know thyself. Ignore this at your own peril, which you do every time you follow someone else's scheme without asking how *you* fit into the equation. "Look to the host"—the host is *you*. Learn this lesson well and not only will you be able to lose weight, maybe for the first time, but you will be well on your way to a life that's bigger and greater and more powerful than you ever imagined.

Picking a Diet: The Critical Missing Step

One day I walked through a torrential downpour to Sparr's drugstore to get my first stethoscope. I was filled with excitement and pride—the stethoscope symbolized the reality of my dream of becoming a doctor.

"Which is the best stethoscope?" I asked the pharmacist.

"It depends on who's listening," he answered.

—*MATTHEW BUDD, M.D.,*
YOU ARE WHAT YOU SAY

Some years ago I was giving a seminar at Equinox Fitness Clubs in New York City, and a young woman got up to ask a question. She was about five feet two inches and considerably overweight; she had a lovely manner and her physical presence radiated "strong midwestern farming stock." She was fair-skinned with freckles, and very articulate.

She was also very frustrated.

"I just do not understand it," she began. "My boyfriend is absolutely gorgeous. He's about six feet tall and muscular, and he has no body fat on him. We eat exactly the same things, we're both on the same low-fat diet, we both are careful about what we eat, and yet I keep gaining weight and he looks like a Calvin Klein ad!"

So I told the woman about my friends Chris and Maria.

Chris and Maria were a married couple who thought it would be a cool thing to take a martial arts class together. Martial arts, they had been told, builds physical power, improves your self-confidence, teaches you patience and serenity and creates inner calm. Meanwhile, you get to walk down the streets with a lot more confidence and in a lot better shape. Eager to start, they entered the dojo.

But they neglected to pay attention to a couple of differences between them.

Maria was 103 pounds. While she had done some gymnastics in high school, and was pretty fast and flexible, she had never lifted weights and wasn't very powerful. Psychologically she was a lot less aggressive than Chris and given her druthers would tend to shy away from a confrontation rather than pursue it to the point where it got ugly. She was a very spiritual woman who liked things like yoga classes and was interested in meditation. Chris, on the other hand, was a big guy who played football in college, had very strongly developed legs, was aggressive in business and was psychologically fearless. While he wasn't a bully, he was also no shrinking violet and had never been known to shy away from a potential encounter. And he loved to win.

Now there must be several hundred schools of martial arts, each with its own strengths, weaknesses and other characteristics. Let's say our couple looks in the phone book and randomly picks a school for tae kwon do, a very aggressive form of karate that involves lots of kicking and strikes and encourages students to begin practice combat almost from the beginning. Who do you think is going to like this method better? Chris or Maria? Who is going to thrive here and who is going to tank?

Or let's say they happen to choose a school for the Wing Chun method. Wing Chun, no less deadly than tae kwon do, was invented by a Buddhist nun named Ng Mui about 300 years ago in southern China and named for her first student, a 100-pound woman named Yim Wing Chun. It is an exquisite martial art (Bruce Lee was a master), but it was developed on the lighter, more flexible body of a woman and uses the opponent's strength and power against him. In addition, Wing Chun has a particular spiritual bent that adds to the effectiveness of the training of its disciples. Who is going to be the A student in *this* class?

Which method is going to be better for Chris? Which for Maria?

Remember, now, I'm not asking you which martial arts form is better. Both will ultimately produce the same results—the ability to kick butt. But they're going to take very different approaches to getting there and there is going to be a significant difference in the fit of each of these methods with each of these two very different individuals.

Just as Chris and Maria belonged in different martial arts classes, the woman in my seminar and her boyfriend needed different *strategies* to maintain lean healthy bodies. This lovely woman was frustrated because she still believed there was such a thing as the "right" diet and she assumed that once she found it, it would produce the same results for both her and her boyfriend. *Wrong.* The strategy they had come up with was working great for her boyfriend, but not so great for her.

See, when you begin to think of diets (yes, I hate that word, too, but let's agree to use it for the time being) as *strategies*, the whole issue of weight loss takes on a different look. A military general formulating a strategy for attack would be idiotic not to take into account the size of his army, the strength of the opposing forces, the climate conditions under which they would be doing battle, the level of fatigue and the psychological strengths and weaknesses of his men and probably a dozen other factors that generals have to think about. A coach formulating a strategy for a sports team does the same thing. She doesn't blindly follow a game plan—she takes into account the strengths of her players, she evaluates the players on the opposing team, she looks at the kind of playing field they're on, she considers any injuries that may have been sustained on either side—and then, if she's a good coach, she adjusts her strategy accordingly. To do otherwise would be folly.

Yet that's exactly how we approach dieting. Someone comes out with a new book, we hear about it through the grapevine, we see the author on television, we read about the diet in a magazine, and we blindly jump in, following some strategy that may have absolutely nothing to do with who we are or the way we live our lives or our individual metabolic constitution. No wonder we're frustrated. We've skipped the critical first step that any athlete, any army, any competitor, any business executive *must* do before jumping into battle: *Understand your team, and understand your competition*. Only then can you devise a strategy that has a chance of working.

The Shape Up plan is a course in how to devise a strategy for weight loss (and improved health in the bargain) that works for *you*. You're the home team in this game, and to devise a successful strategy we need to look at all the players on your field. We have to understand the many factors that go into making each of us metabolically and biochemically unique, so that we can use those factors to best advantage. We need to know what we've got to work with, and we need to fully understand what we're up against.

Strategies are based on assumptions. We assume our opponent is going to behave a certain way—in business, in a boxing ring, on a playing field, on a chess board—and we act in a way that we think will be most effective based on the assumptions we believe to be true. Every diet approaches weight loss according to some set of basic principles that are assumed to be true. But if the basic assumptions are wrong, the strategy is going to tank. That's why we'll be spending a lot of time in this book questioning some of those conventional basic assumptions about weight loss that have been around longer than they deserve to be. You *may* just discover that you've been basing your weight loss strategies on "traditional wisdom" that is actually neither nor wise.

And speaking of traditional wisdom . . .

Virtually every time I speak anywhere, I'm asked some version of the following question: "Why can't you guys make up your minds? First we hear that butter is bad for you, and we should switch to margarine; now we're hearing the opposite. First I'm told cereal and a banana and orange juice is the way to go for breakfast, now you're telling me it's not. Why can't you guys get it together?"

I'll tell you why not.

Nutrition, as a science, is pretty darn young. To put it in perspective, if you condense the entire three-million-year history of mankind into one twenty-four–year period, then nutrition as a science began . . . can you guess?

Three seconds ago.

A mite young to be having all the answers at this point in time, don't you think?

See, in other areas of fitness we don't have this problem. No big debates in the field of anatomy. It's generally accepted where the organs are, the bones, tendons and muscles. And though there's an occasional small squabble about the best way to perform an exercise, the bulk of the information about what muscles move what bones in what direction is pretty much agreed upon.

But this nutrition thing.... Here's a hotbed area that encompasses information about metabolism, habit, psychology, enzymes, hormones, digestion, immune system, history, genetics, race.... And those are just the variables everyone agrees on. Add to that the more controversial issues like insulin insensitivity, leptin receptivity, candida, thyroid underactivity, stress, blood type, food sensitivities, nutrient status, leaky gut, metabolic type and the role of neurotransmitters and, well, you should be getting the picture.

It's not a field ripe for an ecumenical council.

I understand the frustration of hearing different points of view on everything from protein to carbohydrates, dairy to sugar, calories to fat grams, butter to margarine. It's particularly hard when all you want to do is eat right, and no one seems to agree on what "right" means. And you'd prefer not to make a career out of researching every little dispute, especially when it seems like the folks who have made careers out of it aren't doing much better than you in the consensus department.

OK, that's the bad news.

The good news is this: Provided you're willing to take the journey and do some experimenting you can actually discover some really interesting stuff about yourself. Just like every other journey of self-discovery that you've embarked on in your life, you may learn some things that surprise you, that fly in the face of conventional wisdom. But if you are willing to hang out with different points of view, use some critical thinking to evaluate what might make sense, try some things that you might not have tried before and, above all, develop your sense of self-observation, you might learn volumes about what makes you tick.

What foods disagree with you? What foods give you energy? Which ones make you tired? Which ones make you bloated? Which seem to affect your moods, and in what ways? What proportions of carbohydrate, fat and protein seem to make sense for you?

Sounds pretty empowering, doesn't it?

And if you really listen, you might learn about even more than food.

You might learn something about the process of self-discovery.

The History of Dieting: Choosing Strategies

In 1980, when *Consumers Guide* published "Rating the Diets," there were well over 100 diet books for their consideration. With few exceptions the underlying concept was always this: Eat less. Whatever gimmick the authors sold, they were all buying the same underlying theory: Excess calories make you fat.

In 1979 a man named Nathan Pritikin published *The Pritikin Program for Diet and Exercise,* a program that was aimed at reversing heart disease. This book could reasonably be considered the birth of low-fat mania. Suddenly there was a shift in emphasis from just plain calories to calories that specifically came from fat. Pritikin followers were fanatical in their avoidance of fat of any kind and were expected to keep to a puritanical and pristine regimen that kept fat at a ridiculous 10 percent of the diet, was relatively low in protein and emphasized grains. The heir to this throne today is Dean Ornish, a man whom I respect tremendously for his advocacy of the position that love and intimacy and spirituality impact health in far greater ways than we ever imagined, but whose nutritional information is from the dark ages.

During the 1980s and 90s, all manner of low-fat diets prevailed. Fat was the new demon, and an industry was created pandering to our fear and misunderstanding of it. Snackwell low-fat cookies actually surpassed Oreos as America's favorite cookie for a while. For those "in the know," fat in any form at all was about as welcome on the menu as an anarchist at the Republican Governors Association Conference. Pasta and bagels, solely on the basis of their having virtually no fat content, became touted as health foods, which is a little like promoting *the Godfather* as a role model because he liked to play with his grandkids.

Around this time the specialty of "sports nutrition" began to emerge, with spokespeople like Nancy Clark, R.D., and Ellen Coleman, R.D. Ms. Clark is the author of the best-selling *Sports Nutrition Guidebook,*[1] essentially a propaganda piece for the high-carbohydrate diet. I attended one of Ms. Clark's seminars, and my impression was that she, like many of her colleagues in the American Dietary Association, was woefully out of touch with what was happening in clinical nutrition and desperately clinging to an increasingly hard-to-defend party line on such matters as the food pyramid, supplements and the American diet. These folks were basically saying that if people were fat, it was because they ate too many calories and because too many of those calories came from fat. Period. Their answer for weight loss—a very low-fat, high-carbohydrate diet. Their answer for sports nutrition—a very low-fat, high-carbohydrate diet. Their answer for health for all people? You guessed it.

A very low-fat, low-protein, high-carbohydrate diet.

These folks recommended—and continue to recommend—dairy for everyone, grains and cereals, pasta and bread; they lumped fats and sugars together as something to be used "very occasionally." Protein got the lowest percentage of the recommendation pie, clocking in at between 12 and 15 percent of the recommended diet.

If you're reading this book, chances are very good that that very diet made you fat or is preventing you from losing weight. And it's almost certainly not making you any healthier.

Now if you've spent any time around gyms you may be asking, "but what about bodybuilders? *They're* certainly lean, and they eat *plenty* of carbs." And you'd have a point. In fact, the typical bodybuilding diet is almost fanatically low-fat and high-carb (and also, incidentally, *very* high in protein). Anyone who has ever been around a hard-core gym has seen these guys and gals with their Tupperware containers of chicken and rice, or tuna and potatoes. What's up with that?

Well, the simple answer is this: You're not them. Bodybuilders are people whose job it is to be as muscular and lean as possible, and who spend hours a day working at it at a level of intensity most of us will never experience. They are also genetically gifted individuals and—let's get real—many of them use other "tools" to assist them in attaining superhuman leanness. They are *not* the model for the average person, and they are *most certainly* not you and me; although a very high-calorie, low-fat diet may in fact work well for them, it is highly unlikely that it will work well for you and me.

Running parallel to this high-carbohydrate, low-fat roller derby was another river of thought that took a very different approach to weight loss. This approach, mainly associated in the popular press with Robert Atkins, called attention to the body's hormonal response to a high-carbohydrate diet. Atkins was one of the first—though certainly not the last—to point out the enormous role of insulin on the playing field of weight gain (though it was left to his successors to point out its negative role in other health issues). The Atkins diet is very low in carbohydrates, and is designed to trigger a particular state in the body called "ketosis," which happens when carbohydrate intake is very, very small (typically 20–30 grams a day or less, a tiny amount). Ketosis is a kind of forced burning of your fat stores, albeit an incomplete cycle, but one that definitely gets the engines running.

Ketosis is neither as dangerous as its opponents claim and probably not as completely benign in the long haul as its defenders believe. It is something that is safe in the short term if you are not in one of three categories: pregnant, a type 1 diabetic or someone with existing kidney problems. It does not *cause* those conditions (pregnancy, type 1 diabetes and kidney problems), despite the misguided warnings of many orthodox doctors.

I'm often asked what I think of Atkins. Here's my answer: He's a pioneer who became a pariah in traditional medicine and yet continues to ask provocative and important questions about conventional recommendations for diet and supplements that the medical and nutritional establishment does not answer well. He has given us wonderful essays on complementary medicine and has been outspoken in advocating the incorporation of vitamins and minerals to treat conditions that are now only being treated with drugs. His recent work attempts to correct the misconception that he is "against" all carbohydrates.

More recently two charming and frighteningly knowledgeable M.D.s, Michael and Mary Dan Eades, co-wrote the book *Protein Power,* which also uses the concept of low-carbohydrate eating for the purpose of bringing out-of-control insulin levels into balance. The Eadeses do a great job of integrating current information about the best kinds of fats, the best kinds of protein and the best kinds of carbs into their eating plan. (They are also very user-friendly—if you want to show their plan to your doctor, they're very forthcoming about providing research that supports their theory, and they include a "For Your Doctor" section in their book.) For the Eadeses it's not just about what you keep *out* of the diet, but about the quality of what you let *in.* The first stage of the Eades program, like the "Induction" phase of the Atkins plan, will put you in ketosis.

My Shape Up plan, however, is *not* a ketogenic program. You will almost certainly not be in ketosis by eating according to the Shape Up guidelines. Most people do not need to go that far in order to reap the many benefits of lower-carbohydrate eating.

In the vacuum between the lower-carb routines of the Eadeses and the very high-carb regimens of Ornish and Pritikin entered a man who has probably been more misrepresented, misquoted and inadequately credited for his work than anyone in the diet "industry" since Atkins—Dr. Barry Sears. Along with the wonderful Ann Louise Gittleman, former director of the Pritikin Center, Dr. Sears with his *Zone* books suggested a rethinking of the word "balance"; Sears and Gittleman recommended "balanced eating," all right, but redefined "balance" as it ought to have been defined in the first place—not as the unbalanced high-carbohydrate diet of the American Dietetic Association, but as a much more equal distribution among the three major macronutrients—fat, protein and carbohydrates. The 40/30/30 plan (please note that the 40 percent lion's share of the distribution refers to *carbohydrates*, making it maddening that doctors and dietitians continue to misrepresent this as a low-carbohydrate plan) has begun to have a very great influence on the nutritional powers that be, although the speed at which these innovations are being adapted by mainstreamers is glacially slow. The 40/30/30 plan takes the position that an imbalance between insulin and its sister hormone glucagon is at the heart of the matter of getting fat, and that only an eating program that controls insulin levels has a hope of making people both healthier and leaner.[2]

I tend to agree with this approach. The main differences between, for example, the Zone and the Shape Up program is not so much in theory, but in practice and application. The Zone can be a fiendishly difficult program to follow and requires very complicated and exact computations about the proportion of carbohydrates, fat and protein at every meal. In addition, as I'm sure Dr. Sears would agree, there are going to be many people for whom 40 percent of carbohydrates is actually *too* much—and there may be some people for whom it's not enough (I haven't *met* many, but I'm sure they're out there). The Shape Up program helps you figure out where you personally fall on this spectrum.

Is the Shape Up program a "no-carb" diet?

Absolutely not. The Shape Up program is, however, a *no junk* diet (at least most of the time), and unfortunately the vast majority of our carbohydrate intake also happens to be junk.

In my opinion the amount of carbs needed for good health is far less than supporters of the food pyramid and purveyors of traditional dietary information would have you believe. Remember that of the three macronutrients—carbohydrates, protein and fat—the only one you have no physiological need for is carbohydrates. Just for the record, you will die without protein, and you will die without fat. You can live just fine without carbohydrates, though I am certainly not suggesting you do any such thing. (In fact, even the Atkins diet doesn't recommend that you eat no carbs.) I *am* going to recommend that you be very selective in your carb intake and that you get your carbs from high-fiber vegetables, low-sugar fruits and a limited number of good starches and legumes used sparingly and intelligently (oatmeal, sweet potatoes and beans are good examples).

The Shape Up plan recognizes the enormous effect of insulin on your weight-loss efforts. Bringing insulin levels under control is a major goal of the Shape Up plan, but we do it in a somewhat different way. Recognizing the huge variation that exists among people biochemically, metabolically and psychologically, we are going to make suggestions for strategies that are designed to lower your blood sugar and create a balanced hormonal state in which insulin does not behave as the villain it's capable of being. Some of those suggestions may work better for you than others—some may be more realistic, some may just feel better. This is *your* program, and you're going to ultimately have to be the judge of what strategy you can live most comfortably with. Our insulin responses—indeed our entire metabolic wiring for carbohydrate disposal—is very individual, and what may stimulate fat gain in one person is "under the bar" for fat gain in another. We're going to look at the effect different foods have on you and then decide if it makes sense *as a strategy* to include those foods all of the time, some of the time, rarely or never. It's going to be different in every case.

Together we can figure out what's best for *your* case.

But first, let's fry up a few sacred cows and see what kind of burgers they make.

"Everything I Needed to Know About Nutrition I Learned From the Cavemen"

There's no such thing as the healthy diet.

Hey, gotcha!

You thought I said there's no such thing as *a* healthy diet, and that grabbed your attention, didn't it? But I said something entirely different, though no less deserving of your attention. I said there's no such thing as *the* healthy diet, despite the constant efforts of the diet dictocrats to convince you otherwise. That's right. Throughout the world, and throughout history, there have been people who have absolutely thrived eating high-protein, high-fat diets (the Eskimos of Greenland), and there have been people who have absolutely thrived eating low-protein, high-carbohydrate diets (the Bantu of South Africa), and there are people who have thrived eating virtually everything in between.

Once you understand this concept—and I mean really *get* it—you can be free from the dictatorship of the health professionals and other "experts" and you can begin to really seek out the best dietary plan for *you*.

And the best place to start is by looking at what we humans were meant to eat.

The nutritionist Patrick Quillan has a great term for this: He calls it the "factory-specified" diet. Here's what it means: Squirrels eat nuts. It's their factory-specified diet. If there are no nuts around, they can probably survive on other stuff, but they are nut-eating machines and run best on the fuel they adapted to over however many years squirrels have been on the planet: nuts. Think about it. Every time you buy a car, or a Walkman, or a dishwasher, the manufacturer usually gives you some idea of what kind of gas, or batteries, or soap to use *with* the product to get the best performance from it. That's the factory-specified fuel for your machine, it's the one they tested it on in the factory, the one they fine-tuned it to run best on.

So what is the factory-specified diet for humans? How do we find it?

The overriding purpose of every living thing on this planet is to reproduce and perpetuate its species. Every creature on the earth has one major biological purpose and that's to make sure there are other creatures like him that are left on the planet to continue on when he's no longer with us. In every species, including humans, some characteristics are better suited to ensuring that survival of the species than others, and some characteristics are definitely a hindrance. For example, the chameleon that is able to swiftly change colors to blend in to the environment is much more likely to survive and pass on his genes. If there was a chameleon who couldn't do that, chances are he'd get eaten by a predator, so his chances of passing on that defective "can't change color" gene are considerably reduced. The caribou who is weak or blind is more likely to be caught by a wolf and therefore less likely to pass on the genes for blindness or weakness. This isn't to say that nature doesn't throw us curve balls, and that there aren't wonderful miraculous examples of people and animals who were born with "handicaps" and went on to achieve great inspirational heights, it's just to say that as an overall survival strategy, nature seems to make sure that those creatures with the best ability overall to adapt to the environment are the ones that have the best chance of surviving and breeding and therefore passing on their genetic inheritance.

And we, good people, are no different. To figure out what *our* factory-specified diet is, the logical place to look first is the environment we adapted to over the course of a couple of million or so years. And the food supply that environment provided. We too, like all other living creatures, have a factory-specified diet, just like your car has factory-specified gas.

Can your car run on a lesser quality of gas? Sure, probably. Will it run as well? No. Can a squirrel live on meat, or a rabbit on asparagus or a bear on canned peas? Maybe. Will it be living its optimal life? No. Why? Because hundreds of thousands of years of adaptation have crafted its digestive system to best allow it to thrive on the food that its environment is *most likely* to provide; and that's the food on which it is designed to "run best."

Guess what?

It's no different for humans.

Food isn't the only thing this applies to. The skin of people of Nordic descent is not suited to tropical climates—it *is* well-suited to the colder, less sunny climate to which they adapted over thousands of years. As a result, they are extremely sun-sensitive, and they do not tan well if at all. On the other hand, Africans, Mediterraneans and anyone whose ancestors lived for millennia in the tropics have skin that produces a lot of melanin; they are therefore much more protected and much less likely to burn under the same conditions that would fry a Norseman. Why? *Because hot sun is a condition under which they normally live and to which they have adapted.*

Eskimos have adapted to their "normal" environmental conditions of extremely bitter cold by developing more body fat. They also thrive on a diet of primarily meat and fat—caribou, moose and seal constituting the bulk of their calories, precisely the food sources that are most abundant in their environment. Hawaiians, on the other hand, thrive on a diet of fruit and coconut and fish (the Tokelauans of Polynesia, incidentally, eat a high-fat diet of about 63 percent coconut and have virtually no heart disease). The Pima Indians have a "thrifty" gene that allows them to survive and thrive in the desert on their very low-calorie native diet. But take them out of their native environment, put them on the reservation and give them access to unlimited mini-marts in downtown Arizona cities, and you witness the epidemic of diabetes and obesity that has been their fate since World War II. Hundreds of years of successful adaptation to the food found in the arid desert have made them supremely unsuited to the food found in the local 7-Eleven.

Ever wonder why they tell Americans not to drink the water in Mexico, but the Mexicans who live there seem to have no problem with it? Now you know why.

Adaptation.

Take a ski lift to the top of a mountain during the summer months and you'll see an example of this kind of adaptation for yourself. Every half-mile or so, there will be an enormous change in the kind of wild vegetation that you see as you ascend the mountain. Plants that thrive in the lower altitude where they are exposed to warmer temperatures and more water do not survive in the higher, more rarified atmospheres where it's cold and dry, and vice versa. Hundreds, or thousands, of years of adaptation to natural environmental conditions allowed plants with a hardiness for cold to "pass on" this survival trait and thrive under cold or barren conditions, while plants with an affinity for warmer, wetter conditions do great at the lower altitudes but die out at the higher ones.

Now here's the point—please, as the great writer William Goldman says, *tattoo this behind your eyelids*:

The human genus has been on the planet for 2.5 million years. Modern humans have existed from somewhere between 100,000 and 300,000 years. *There is absolutely no reason to assume that in all that time there has been any substantial change in our digestive systems and nutritional needs.*

In other words, it's not our plumbing that's changed, it's the food supply.

C. Leigh Broadhurst, Ph.D., author of *Diabetes: Prevention and Cure*, puts it in perspective for us: "Virtually all of us lived in Africa 50,000 years ago; races evolved 30,000 years ago; the last glaciers receded and agriculture developed 10,000 years ago; and McDonald's arrived 100 years ago."

Given that, on what should we base our dietary guidelines?

The apologists for a food industry that has existed in its present form for less than a blip on the radar screen of human development? Or the diet of humankind for the last two million years?

As hunter-gatherers, we ate the following: things we could hunt, fish, catch, dig up or gather. And furthermore, things that were likely to be found in our immediate universe, not trucked in from a distant area and put on a shelf in a supermarket with a preservative that would allow it to sit there for six months without spoiling. We ate, and adapted to, *natural* foods, and natural foods meant, simply, whatever was around us, in season, freshly hunted, caught or harvested.

Which means, depending on where you came from and where you lived, some combination of meat, fish, and vegetation. (The combinations and proportions were different for different people, but the basic buffet was the same.) Here's what we did *not* eat until fairly recently in human history: the products of agriculture (which was developed only 10,000 years ago, and not adopted by many until much later); a high proportion of grains; lots of dairy (there are exceptions; read on) and anything that spoiled easily or couldn't be preserved naturally. We ate traditional, nourishing fats, proteins and, believe it or not, very few carbohydrates.

How do we know this?

We know it from the excellent studies of the remaining hunter-gatherer societies that existed well into the twentieth century, isolated from industrial centers. We know it from the superb work of such pioneers as Dr. Loren Cordain in the field of nutritional anthropology. We know it because anthropologists have been able to determine, from ingenious studies of fossils and bones and teeth marks, precisely what people ate for eons prior to the arrival of modern food-processing techniques and from excellent data showing how those people lived and what diseases they did—and did not—contract.

Now when I talk about humankind and the food we were designed to live on, is that going to be the same for everyone?

Well, funny you should ask.

At the beginning of this century, one of the most profoundly important studies in the history of nutrition was undertaken by a man named Weston Price. Dr. Price was a dentist and was interested in finding out more about why dental disease was so rampant in civilized nations. But like many great pioneers, he accidentally discovered a lot more than he was looking for and in the process has given us some of the most important data about human nutrition ever assembled.

Dr. Price investigated fourteen tribes. He journeyed to remote areas that were completely dependent on their own resources for food. These areas were isolated from developing urban centers and in many ways were untouched by civilization. In most cases Dr. Price was also able to compare people who lived on their native diets ("isolated" tribespeople) with members of the same tribe who had ventured into the cities and whose lifestyle and diet had changed accordingly ("modernized" tribespeople). He investigated isolated and modernized Swiss, Irish, Eskimos, North American Indians, Melanesians, Polynesians, African tribes, Australian Aborigines, Torres Strait Islanders, New Zealand Maori, and Peruvian Indians. Anyone who has ever seen his photographs comparing representative members of these groups will not soon forget them. In virtually every photograph of the isolated tribesmen, the teeth look like an American toothpaste ad. They're strong, white and even, the facial bones are beautiful and symmetrical, the skin glows and the faces radiate good health and cheer. The modernized tribespeople, on the other hand, have uneven, missing and decaying teeth, rot in their mouth and gums, facial and bone deformities and an overall look that can't be mistaken for anything but general unhealthiness.

What can we conclude from these remarkable studies? Was there some magical, terrific food that all of these primitive or isolated hunter-gatherer societies ate that kept them relatively disease free? Absolutely not. The diets of the healthy primitives studied by Dr. Price were extremely heterogeneous. Some were high in animal products, some were not; some were high in sea , some were not; the isolated Swiss practically lived on fresh cream and raw milk direct from the cow; others contained no dairy whatsoever. Some diets contained almost no plant foods; some contained a huge number of fruits, vegetables and grains. Some groups ate primarily cooked foods; others ate a higher proportion of raw food. But here's the kicker: Not one of these primitive diets contained *any* refined foods. There was no white sugar, no flour, no canned goods, no skimmed milk, no refined oils, no partially hydrogenated *anything*. The only preserving that went on was drying, salting and fermenting, all of which, when done by hand, preserve the nutrients in food and may even increase them.

Dr. Price believed that the primitive people had some "innate wisdom," that they intuitively knew something we "civilized" people didn't know, but on this point he may have been wrong. As the great Dr. Abram Hoffer, M.D., Ph.D., points out in his foreword to the fifth edition of Price's book,

> There [was] no *innate wisdom* because, until chemistry was discovered and applied to food technology, there was *no need for it*. Early peoples had little choice but to *eat foods that they had adapted to, for no other food was available.* The local animals, fish, whole grains, vegetables, some fruits and nuts provided a limited choice. They could not browse in supermarkets containing 15,000 items of which 90 percent, or perhaps more, are junk. If primitive peoples had obtained their food from a supermarket, they would have consumed as much junk as do high-tech peoples. (emphasis mine)

In other words, these primitive people were eating their factory-specified diet. They were eating the foods they had adapted to eating, the foods they were supposed to eat, the ones that were found in their immediate environment, the ones they could catch, hunt for, gather, pluck or dig up, and they were eating them in pretty much their fresh and natural state. What they were *not* doing was going to the supermarket and choosing from a dazzling array of processed, refined, denatured food products that had long since lost any of their nutritional value, had been pulverized and processed into oblivion, and then colored and sweetened and preserved beyond recognition so they could sit on the shelf without spoiling while their manufacturers devised brilliant ad campaigns to tell you how healthy and delicious they were and to make you feel that living without them was a life of deprivation.

Now obviously we can't all go back to Eden. But we can learn something about the factory-specified diet for humanity from these studies. And the take-home point is this: *There is no one healthy diet.* But *all* healthy diets have certain things in common and you can ultimately devise the best strategy by following these principles:

- The more you can mimic eating what you would have eaten in the wild, the better.
- The closer your food looks to the way it is found in nature, the better.
- The less stuff you eat that comes in packages, the better.
- The longer the *shelf* life, the worse it is for *your* life.
- The less stuff you eat with ingredients you can't pronounce, the better.

And this leads us to the first—and maybe most important—lesson to be learned from studying the history of dieting. We learn it not from studying the dietary wisdom of the last twenty or thirty years, but from studying the dietary wisdom of the ages. Memorize it and remember it for it will serve you well in devising your best eating strategy.

The more food you eat that could have been grown, hunted, fished for, caught, plucked or gathered, the better off you'll be.

Notes

1. Ms. Coleman recently published *The Ultimate Sports Nutrition Handbook*. Same song, different key.

2. There were other people who weighed in with terrific programs that recognized the importance of insulin in getting fat. Dr. Diana Schwarzbein, whose "Schwarzbein Principle" is always on my recommended list, took her version of the lower carbohydrate diet to market, and one of the earlier pioneers in recognizing the role of commercial breads and pastas and other high-insulin-producing foods in making us fat was Cliff Sheats with his "Lean Body" program in the 1980s. Drs. Richard and Rachel Heller, who took a still different approach, also made a contribution, as did Dr. Carlon Colker with is "Greenwich Diet."

CALORIES AND HORMONES

The Tyranny of the Calorie

**When you cannot express it in numbers,
your knowledge is of a meager and unsatisfactory kind.**

—LORD KELVIN (STATING "THE STATISTICIAN'S DICTUM")

Get a life!

—JONNY BOWDEN

In the late 1800s a chemist named Wilbur Atwater invented the calorie.

Well, to be exact, he didn't exactly invent it. What he did was discover that there was an objective way to measure the energy value of food. By putting food in a device which is now called a "bomb calorimeter" and basically torching it and measuring the ash, he could determine how much energy was being released into the air and therefore estimate how much energy was actually contained within the molecular bonds of the food itself. The calorie itself is a measure of heat—to be precise, one calorie is the amount of heat it takes to raise the temperature of one liter of water from thirteen degrees dentigrade to fourteen degrees centigrade. Scientists figure out the amount of calories in food by burning it. When the food burns, the chemical bonds break, releasing energy in the form of heat. The amount of heat given off is a direct measure of the food's energy value (i.e., how many calories it has).

Chemists now had a way of quantifying exactly how much food—or energy—was being taken in during a meal. Within a decade, they realized that it was also possible to apply the currency of calories to energy being expended by the human body in various activities, from sleeping to running. They now had an objective measure of energy input from food, plus an objective measure of energy output from exercise and activity.

And the tyranny of the calorie equation was born.

For decades, the prevailing nutritional wisdom was based on what was called the "energy balance" equation: that is, weight stays the same when calories in equals calories out. We take in calories from food; we burn up calories in the process of living. When calories *in* equals calories *out*, weight stays pretty much the same. This theory looks at the body as operating on the same principle as a checkbook. A checkbook has two types of entries: income and expenses. If you *take in* a lot more money than you *spend*, you have a *positive* balance sheet—in essence, you've got extra money and a nice fat savings account. If you *spend* more money than you *take in*, you have a *negative* balance—to pay your bills you have to dig into those savings. When income equals expenses, you have a zero balance. According to the energy balance theory, it works the same way with calories. If calorie "income" (from food) equals calorie "expenses," energy is "balanced" and your weight stays the same. If you eat more calories than you use, those excess calories go into your savings account, which, for most people, is located in the buttocks, thighs or abdominal region. You're taking in more than you're putting out—and you get fat. On the other hand, if you use up more calories than you take in, you dip into that savings account of yours (your fat stores) to pay the bill—and the result is you lose weight.

A nice, neat, compact theory.

And, oh, that it were so simple.

Part of the problem with this theory is our infatuation with measurement. We tend to believe what we can measure. Give a bunch of scientists a tool that lets them measure something objectively, and you can count on the fact that in short order that measurement tool will take on a life of its own, become an icon, and before you know it you'll have a religion of true believers on your hands. The less imaginative scientists—and believe me, there are plenty of those—will hang on to it for dear life and use it as a substitute for thinking. Before long, it will become dogma. Entire cottage industries will spring up around it, it will become the standard by which everything is judged, there will be huge economic incentives in keeping the status quo and anyone questioning whether the measurement provides the full picture, or even continues to serve a useful purpose, will be considered a heretic and "anti-scientific." We've seen this in our own time with a dozen different measurement tools: SAT scores, creativity tests, I.Q. tests, cholesterol tests, even the Nielsen ratings for television. Do these things really measure what they're supposed to? Or, more important, *are they giving us complete or even useful information about that which they are supposed to be enlightening us?*

Take cholesterol. Cholesterol is turning out to be a very unreliable predictor of heart disease. People with perfectly fine cholesterol levels have heart attacks, and plenty of people with highly elevated levels don't. A recent study in *Circulation* showed that the ratio of triglycerides to HDL predicts heart disease *sixteen times better* than cholesterol readings. After twenty-five years during which he was exiled into scientific purgatory for daring to question cholesterol dogma, Killmer McCullough has finally been recognized by mainstream medicine for demonstrating the tremendous association between the levels of a compound in the body called homocysteine and heart attacks, an association far more important than the one between cholesterol and heart attacks, and a connection that was derided by the cholesterol establishment for decades. (You can be sure this concept has made it to mainstream when you see television ads for Centrum vitamins touting the products ability to "lower homocysteine levels.") We now know that even the so-called (and unfortunately named) "bad" cholesterol is made up of several different fractions, and that only one of these (LDLb) is really likely to cause any damage. And, to top it off, we have *overwhelming* evidence that in any event *dietary* cholesterol has very little effect on *serum* cholesterol levels and negligible effect on health. Even Ansel Keys, whose highly flawed "Seven Countries" study gave birth to the whole cholesterol madness in the first place, has said, "Dietary cholesterol has no effect on blood cholesterol. We've known that right along." Yet tell that to the multibillion-dollar industry that markets "no-cholesterol" foods to the public, and to orthodox docs who continue to recommend low-cholesterol diets as the best way to protect the heart.

Remember this well when you continue to hear the old guard defend their nutritional and medical sacred cows: The establishment changes direction about as easily and quickly as a thirty-five-ton oil steamer.

So we continue to hear that the only thing that matters in weight loss is calories. "A calorie is a calorie is a calorie" say these Gertrude Steins of medicine. The only thing that makes you lose weight is when you eat fewer calories than you burn up. When confronted with the anecdotal and clinical experience of thousands of people whose experience would indicate that it's a lot more complex than that, they sneer and state a conceptual catch-22: *People who lose weight on a diet that doesn't count calories only did so because the "fad" diet they were on must have been in actuality a low calorie diet.*

I'm not so sure.

The human body contains literally thousands of enzymes, eicosanoids, hormones, neurotransmitters and other compounds that operate on or are affected by food and its metabolic by-products in the journey from entrance to exit. To assume that this pathway is identical in every human being, and that the incredibly complex process of weight gain, weight loss and energy production happens exactly the same way in every single person and can be quantified by simply measuring what goes in and what comes out without taking into account what goes on inside the individual human body, seems to me a preposterously short-sighted and limited view of human metabolism.

Now, you might get the idea from what I've been saying that I think that calories have nothing important to tell us and that the calorie balance theory of weight loss is useless.

That's not entirely correct.

I don't think the information given us by calories in/calories out is useless. I *do* think it's very incomplete. And I do think, with one exception which we'll talk about in Chapter 18 ("It's a War Out There"), calorie counting is *not* the best strategy for weight loss.

Calories are one way of measuring the total amount of food we're putting into our bodies, and it certainly doesn't hurt to be conscious of them, but in no way does the calories in/calories out theory present a true and complete picture of what happens when we eat food and gain or lose weight. There are simply far too many individual variations to predict how much of that food we eat will efficiently turn into energy and be burned off as heat and how much of it will end up mocking and tormenting us as it takes up residence on our bodies and expands our waistlines and stretches our pants.

Am I saying that calories don't count at all? No, I'm not. What I am saying is that they no longer deserve top billing on the marquee of weight loss.

And by the way, it's the same deal with exercise. Do you buy into those calorie readouts on the exercise machines you've been pumping away on at the gym? Forget it. Not only are they notoriously inaccurate at best, not only do they overestimate calories expended (think they would sell as many machines if they told you what was really happening?), but they are notoriously bad at factoring in the myriad of individual variations that occur when different people get on the same machine. When I taught personal training at New York's Equinox Fitness Clubs, we had an exercise physiology lab that contained an apparatus called a metabolic cart. You would get on a treadmill and put on a mask attached to a computer that would measure your oxygen intake and your carbon dioxide output at different levels of exercise intensity. Then the computer would calculate your caloric expenditure as you exercised. *The individual variations were absolutely astonishing, and they would often vary enormously from what the standard equations would predict.*

Look, suppose I rented a car in Los Angeles and wanted to buy just enough gas to get to San Diego. The distance is 120 miles. If I fill the tank and only use a third of it, there's no refund and I will have wasted money, so I want to get a good idea of how much gas to buy. Think about it for a minute before reading further, and see if you can guess the answer to this question: *How many gallons I should purchase?*

OK, give up? Well, yes, it was a trick question. And the trick is this: There's no correct answer unless you have one missing critical piece of information, which I didn't give you. Before you can answer the question of how many gallons of gas I need, you have to answer *another* question: *What kind of car did I rent?*

If I rented a Jeep I might get only ten miles to the gallon, but if I rented a Volkswagen I might get thirty. *And it's the same thing with calories.* As we'll see time and again in this book, we are all metabolically unique. *To assume we all use calories in exactly the same way, with the same efficiency, is tantamount to assuming all cars need the same amount of gas to travel 120 miles.*

The bottom line? We are all biochemically, physiologically unique, and to be successful at weight loss we better stop relying so heavily on general formulas and measurements, no matter how attractive they are, and begin understanding that the real action is in understanding what happens inside that completely unique, special environment that is *you*. Because it's completely different from what happens inside your neighbor, your husband, your co-workers, the person you met who did great on the latest Hollywood diet and anyone else who claims to have found "the answer" in a formula.

Calories *Do* Count—but Don't Count Calories

I tell my clients not to count calories. But saying "don't count calories" is not the same as saying "calories don't count."

Most people will lose weight if they design for themselves an eating strategy using the suggestions in my Shape Up program. Here's why: Most of us are simply eating so badly that by making a concerted effort to reduce the foods on the "B" list while adding more foods that are on the "A" list, we will begin to lose weight. It's as simple as that. Our food supply is so toxic, so wrong for health and vitality and leanness, that simply changing the diet in the direction of the Shape Up guidelines will produce noticeable and positive results (which you'll see not only in your waistline but in your mood and your energy as well). By eating more of the high-fiber, high-volume, nutrient-dense foods and higher amounts of the better fats and proteins and eliminating the sugar-filled, processed, refined, high-carbohydrate junk foods that constitute the bulk of the American diet, you will automatically be making the changes you need to make to change your body, without counting calories. This doesn't mean that calories don't "count"—they do—it just means that experience has shown that if you do the right things, calorie intake will often take care of itself.

There are several other reasons I don't recommend counting calories as a first strategy for fat loss:

1. It's very time consuming (you need a food scale and—more important—you need to use it all the time to be truly accurate).
2. Even then, it's usually impractical (especially if, as most people do today, you eat a good portion of your meals away from home).
3. It can feed into a very obsessive mentality about food—it doesn't *have* to, but it can.
4. It's not fun, and . . .
5. Calorie counting as a strategy tends to feed into the outdated idea that calories are all that matter. It is entirely possible to eat the right number of calories and still not lose weight if you are eating the wrong foods. (Remember, if you eliminate most of the wrong foods and eat more of the right foods, you will begin to see results without having to.)

All over America there are men and women who are able to rattle off the caloric count of absolutely any food in the U.S. Department of Agriculture handbook. But this is like knowing the price of everything and the value of nothing. The *composition* of your calories, as you will see, is *at least* as important as their number, despite what the old-fashioned nutrition "experts" continue to preach.

So to help round out the very incomplete picture of weight loss and weight gain that the calorie balance theory has to offer, we have to begin looking at what happens once food enters the body. How do we become fat? How do we become lean? And why, oh why, do the rules seem to be so different for different people?

A good place to start is with the hormonal response to food.

The Hormonal Response to Food

The great thing, then, in all education, is to make our nervous system our ally instead of our enemy.

— WILLIAM JAMES

Probably the major fault line that separates the old guard in nutrition from the new is the fascinating subject of our hormonal response to food. The old guard insists it has little effect on weight loss and gain (because only calories matter, remember?), while the new guard believes that a program that doesn't take the behavior of hormones into account is doomed to failure. Full disclosure: I think the old guard's nuts.

A juvenile, or type 1, diabetic is fully capable of eating his parents out of house and home, downing five thousand calories a day. If calories were all that mattered, he should be getting fat, right? But he doesn't. In fact, he continues to lose weight at an unexplained and alarming rate, which, coupled with copious amounts of urination and unbearable thirst, is an unmistakable sign of type I diabetes.

Why doesn't he gain weight? Because his pancreas does not produce enough of one of the most important hormones we'll be talking about throughout this book: insulin. And without insulin, the sugar (and amino acids) in his bloodstream cannot get into the cells and be used for either building muscle or fat. Without insulin, he cannot gain weight. Without insulin, in fact, he will die, which was the fate of anyone unlucky enough to have this disease in the early part of the twentieth century, before the role of insulin was fully understood and before it became possible to provide it to those who were missing it.

Interestingly, I was recently interviewed on a radio show by my dear but misguided friend Liz Neporent who is clearly in the camp of the old guard. She said to me: "Look, I simply can't believe this whole theory that insulin has such a big effect on weight. After all, there are dozens of other hormones to consider, why all the emphasis on this one?" That's like saying to a basketball player, "There are so many skills that go into being a well-rounded athlete. Why all this emphasis on how high you can jump?" It's certainly true that many factors need to be taken into account in evaluating all-around athletic ability, but if you're choosing a player for your *basketball* team, his marathon time or his weight-lifting ability is just not a big consideration. On the basketball field, some skills matter more than others. And while it is absolutely true that levels of other hormones can have a profound effect on weight-loss efforts—thyroid hormone, for example, testosterone, estrogen or human growth hormone—on the playing field of weight loss, insulin is the Michael Jordan of hormones.

And there is a drug, widely available, completely legal, which you can use right now to modulate your levels of this all-important hormone. In fact, you probably have it in your home this very minute.

It's called "food."

Look, if food is a drug—and it is—my mission is to teach you how to make it *last* as long as it can and feel as *good* as it can. You were not meant to live your life in a body four times the size of the "blueprint," with flagging energy and low self-esteem, suffering from arthritis, asthma, blood sugar diseases, cancer, heart disease, osteoporosis and all the other maladies that have cropped up like weeds in the last hundred or so years. It's your birthright to live out your life in good health in a strong and fit body, with a strong sense of your own worth and purpose and an ability to contribute and give back to the world—not be riddled with angst about not being perfect because you don't look like the heroin-addicted waif-du-jour on the cover of some fashion glossy. And your individual hormonal response to the food you eat is a big player in the weight loss game, not to mention its effect on your mood, your energy and your sense of well-being.

Your choice of food determines your body's hormonal response to it.

But let's understand how all this works. And in doing so, let's take a look at this hormone insulin and see why it's getting so much attention. Understand this, and a lot of dietary information that you may have been confused about will become clear almost immediately.

When you eat a meal, any meal, your blood sugar rises. The body knows that it needs to keep blood sugar within a healthy range, so in its infinite wisdom it dispatches the hormone insulin to "escort" sugar into the cells, where it can be used for energy, or, all too often, into the adipose tissues, where it is stored as fat. Insulin is known as an "anabolic" hormone, since it is involved in building up the body, mainly the cells which it nurtures with its periodic delivery of the body's building blocks—glucose (sugar), amino acids (protein) and fatty acids (fat).

So the job of insulin is two-fold. One, to get the blood sugar back to normal. Two, to get the sugar (and the fat and the protein) escorted into the cells, where they can be used for energy or where they can be transformed into something we can store for later use. When this system works well, which it sometimes does, everything is fine. However, in response to a continuous high-carbohydrate, low-fat diet that most of us have been taught is healthy and that also happens to contain a ton of sugar, very little fiber and an awful lot of processed food, that's not what happens at all.

What happens is this: We eat a large high-carb meal. Our blood sugar goes skyrocketing. The pancreas says, "Uh, oh, better send in the insulin troops," but now there's so much sugar in the bloodstream that a little bit of insulin isn't enough—we need more to do the job. If you're a sedentary person the situation is worse. Your muscle cells begin to show some resistance to the effects of insulin. They tend to stop answering the door and essentially begin to sing the chorus of that Little Richard song, "I Hear You Knockin' but You Can't Come In!" After a meal, blood sugar stays elevated longer because very few muscle cells will take it in. More insulin is secreted by the poor overworked pancreas in an attempt to get that blood sugar down. Since sugar (and its insulin escort) isn't getting a great reception by the muscle cells, it goes to its second choice—can anyone guess where?

Exactly.

Insulin and its client, sugar, knock on the door of the fat cells, where they find a big old welcome mat. And meanwhile look what's happened elsewhere in the body, none of it good: Blood sugar is perennially high, as are circulating levels of insulin (which, incidentally, puts you at risk for a whole cornucopia of conditions that you do not want). When blood sugar and insulin levels rise precipitously they eventually come down with a crash—and a whole cycle of low and high energy, cravings and weight gain has begun.

And, in the bargain . . .

We get fat.

This situation—in which the cells get progressively less hospitable to the action of insulin and the body becomes more and more likely to store the breakdown products of food as fat is called insulin resistance, and it is at the heart of a condition called Syndrome X, itself a huge risk factor for heart disease and diabetes. In Syndrome X you have perennially high blood sugar; your poor pancreas is working like a dog to put out enough insulin to do its job of keeping blood sugar levels out of the diabetic range, and for a time it's succeeding (though how long it's going to be able to continue to do so is anybody's guess). The debate that rages right now in nutrition circles is about the exact connection between obesity and insulin resistance. Dr. Gerald Reavan, the man who first called attention to Syndrome X and gave it its name in the 1980s, insists that obesity does not cause insulin resistance (though he agrees that it can make it worse). He believes that you can be of normal weight and still be insulin resistant. Other experts feel that obesity and insulin resistance walk hand in hand. In my opinion, what we have here is a classic chicken and egg problem, and one we regular people don't really have to beat our heads against the wall about too much. Here's why: We know that insulin resistance and obesity are very frequently found together. We also know that insulin resistance can be dramatically improved by dietary changes. It's a darn good bet that even if insulin resistance doesn't technically "cause" obesity, it certainly makes it worse; obesity *definitely* makes insulin resistance worse.

Look, people can get fat by eating too much food and not exercising enough, independent of any metabolic disorder. We've always known that. We *also* know that it's a heck of a lot easier for some people to get fat than others and that those who get fat the easiest probably have some degree of insulin resistance. People whose insulin response is completely normal, in my opinion, are the ones who have a shot at losing weight on Weight Watchers, Slim Fast, Jenny Craig and other portion control programs. (How successfully they keep it off is another question entirely.) These people are the best candidates for losing weight by programs that ignore the composition of the food and just reduce its amount, by either special drinks, low-fat diets or calorie control. (There is plenty of evidence that they also gain it back easily, but that's another story.) The problem comes when the entire medical and nutritional establishment tells us that these people represent the entire population and that all anyone has to do to lose weight is watch their portions. If you are one of the lucky ones who got fat just by eating too much food for a bit of time, and your metabolism is in perky working order, good for you. But if you are in that 25 percent of the population that even conservatives agree is seriously insulin insensitive, or in the majority of the population that lies somewhere between optimal insulin sensitivity and total disaster, then low-fat diets and calorie counting just ain't gonna work for you.

The bottom line is this: We want food that produces a balanced hormonal response. We do not want high circulating levels of insulin, which has now been implicated in a devil's quartet of conditions—high blood pressure, high triglycerides, cardiovascular disease and diabetes (chronic high levels of insulin are a *strong* risk factor for type 2 diabetes). Understand that this does not mean that insulin is a bad hormone—you couldn't live without it. The problem is not the insulin, but the lack of balance between insulin and its sister hormone, glucagon. Whereas insulin signals the body to store things (like sugar and, to a lesser extent in very overweight people, the protein of amino acids), its sister pancreatic hormone glucagon has a different effect. When blood sugar is low, glucagon tells the cells to let some out so as to bring blood sugars back up to normal. It's a *releasing* hormone, not a *storage* hormone. We want—we *need*—a balance between the two. A good working relationship.

We don't have one.

And the blame for that imbalance has to be shouldered in large measure by the American Diet, notably the fashionably low-fat, high-carb diet of the 1980s and beyond, the diet the American Dietetic Association and the American Heart Association and the National Cholesterol Education Program continue to recommend shamelessly. It raises blood sugar, which causes insulin to rise, it puts you at risk for a lot of nasty diseases, and—because of the metabolic configuration of most overweight people—it makes it terribly difficult to lose weight.

Here's the take-home point for Shape Uppers:

A diet based on commercial breads, pastas and cereals—such as those recommended for six to eleven servings on the USDA food pyramid—will make most people fat. At the very least, it will make it supremely difficult to lose weight. And if you still don't see what all the fuss is about, consider this basic biochemical fact: The body does not burn fat in the presence of high levels of insulin.

What triggers insulin? Many things. Certainly carbohydrates. To a lesser extent protein, though not nearly to the extent that most carbs do. Large meals—of *any* composition—are a trigger for it (more on this later).

Insulin is also, incidentally, a stimulus for a fat-storing enzyme called lipoprotein lipase. It has been hypothesized that chronically overweight people have very effective and perhaps overactive lipoprotein lipase activity. This certainly can't be helped by eating food that stimulates higher and higher levels of insulin.

What we need instead is to eat food that raises blood sugar slowly, takes it to a comfortable level and keeps it there for a long time. We need our blood sugar—and our corresponding insulin levels—to behave more like a gentle lake than the Atlantic Ocean during hurricane season. And we need food and supplements that provide all the materials to keep our metabolism humming along efficiently and productively. In short, we need food, supplements and exercise in just the right amounts to turn our bodies into lean, mean, fat-burning machines.

And that's what the Shape Up program is about.

GETTING STARTED

Five Things to Do Before Beginning the Program

Just as I asked you to throw out your concept of what a diet is, I want you to throw away your concept of what a *diet book* is. I'm going to ask you to do some things in this program that you may never have done and that you almost *certainly* have not done in connection with losing weight. I need you to trust me on this. Some of the things I'm going to suggest that you do may seem unrelated to weight loss, but they're in this program for a very good reason, maybe the only reason that ultimately matters: *They work.* So for now, turn down the volume on that little voice that may be chattering away in your ear after you read the first assignments, that voice that may be asking things like "What does *that* have to do with getting in shape?" We'll be talking a lot more about that little voice later on. For now, just please ask it to be quiet for a minute while *you* do the homework.

1. Buy a notebook. But not just any notebook. Shop carefully, and find one that really speaks to you in some way. Find one that fits your lifestyle, that you can carry around with you. It's going to be your constant companion for the next eight weeks, a private place to record information, feelings and observations that are very personal to you, so choose something with a texture and a design that you really like.

It's interesting to watch how people go about doing this seemingly easy first step. I've noticed that people who just go to the drugstore and absent-mindedly pick up any old notebook often feel subconsciously that the stuff they're going to be writing in it isn't all that important. I've noticed in my own life that when I just pick up any old standard school notebook from the corner store for a course I'm taking or for a project I'm doing, I don't seem to treat it very seriously. Before long, the book gets dog-eared and ugly and stuffed away in a drawer somewhere. When I go out and buy a really nice book to keep my notes in, I tend to give what goes into that book a lot more care and a lot more attention. I still have my notebooks from the Designs for Health Institute Seminars in Clinical Nutrition right

43

by my desk, beautiful hardbound journals that contain my notes for some of the best seminars and workshops I've ever taken. I refer to them constantly, and they look great sitting on my bookshelf. I believe that the care you take in picking out the right book to keep your notes in will subconsciously influence you to treat this whole journaling process as one that is really significant. And it is. Remember, this journal is a reflection of your life, at least at this point in time. It should reflect the care you are going to put into understanding that life and the issues surrounding your weight. Choose it carefully.

This is a good time to begin listening to your unconscious. If for some reason something red speaks to you, that's what you should buy. Don't analyze it, just do it. If you like the feel of cloth, or leather, or parchment paper, go for it. Part of this program is about understanding and honoring parts of yourself that you may never have explored before. You're going to use this journal as an important tool to learn about your weight, what it means in your life and how to finally take control of it; you're going to develop real, useful tools that can serve and empower you for the rest of your life. The blank journal you buy to hold that information is the vessel of your change and your empowerment. So choose the vessel carefully.

2. Make a list of at least *five ways you could add activity to your daily life.* You don't have to do any of them yet; just think about all the ways you *could*, and then write them down in your new notebook. This is an imagination exercise—be as mundane or as creative as you like. Your list could include such things as parking further from the mall and walking to the entrance, bringing a jump rope to work to use on your lunch hour, climbing the steps to your office or home or doing a few extra minutes of gardening. Feel free to be whimsical. It doesn't matter no one's going to check on you. If one way that occurs to you is to have your husband build you a gym in the garage, put it down on the list, no matter how farfetched it may seem. Have fun with this exercise. Think "out of the box." Imagination is a big part of this program.

The universe can almost always be counted on to present obstacles—actually, I prefer to call them challenges—not just to exercise, but to a host of things you want to do but can never seem to find time for. I don't need to tell you this. And I don't mean to diminish those obstacles. (I can almost hear you saying, "I know where you're going with this, Jonny, but you don't understand. In *my* case, there *really isn't* any time.")

I know, I know. And I know I'm asking you to make a big leap of faith by even suggesting that the act of commitment could actually precede a practical plan. Sort of like deciding you are going to buy a certain house even when you have no idea where the money's gonna come from. But people do it every day. Businesses—even empires—have been started like that. And in some small measure, every one of us can do it.

So here you are, with absolutely no time, a schedule that is packed with job, spouse, kids, soccer, there's no gym in your neighborhood, you have a long commute home and now I'm asking you to commit to do something else.

Listen, Jonny, *you just don't understand*. There's no *time*.

First question. If your doctor suddenly told you, God forbid, that you had a potentially fatal illness and that the only way you could beat it was to sit quietly and meditate for twenty minutes a day. . . what would you do?

OK, now we've gotten the time factor out of the way.

(By the way, I wish I could share with you the number of clients who have come into my office at the point in time when their doctors have read them the riot act, and a lot of the physical damage has already been done. And how they wish they'd paid attention to their health before it got into crisis management mode. And how much they appreciate their lives now that they've had a brush with their own mortality. You don't need to wait for that to happen.)

So now let's say you're ready to play along with me. You still don't believe there's any time, you still think I'm talking to everyone out there *but* you, you still think I don't understand how *truly* busy you are, but you're willing to go along for the ride and make this commitment to your health regardless of the fact that the circumstances seem to be stacked against you.

So.

I want you to make a list of all the times, places and ways that you could fit some kind of physical activity into your day. I'm going to give you a head start with the following questions. Don't look at these and say "but that doesn't apply to me." Some won't apply to you, some may. Doesn't matter. They're only here to give you a head start on your own list.

When you go on a short errand, can you walk instead of taking the car?

Are there stairs in your office or apartment building? Could you climb them for five minutes a day?

Can you walk briskly around your block once before retiring for the night?

Do you take a lunch hour? Could you use twenty to thirty minutes of it to walk, run, stretch, meditate, or do push-ups, crunches, squats, lunges, or dips? Or could you use those stairs (see above)?

If you live in a city, can you get off the subway one stop early and walk the rest of the way to work? (One New York client I had did this, coming and going; we estimated that the short ten-minute walk he took twice a day burned 25,000 calories a year, or a bit more than seven pounds!)

Can you lift weights for fifteen minutes twice a week? (How about on weekends?) No weights? How about push-ups and squats and crunches?

There's an old maxim used in the transformational consciousness movement. You may be familiar with one version of it from the movie *Field of Dreams* ("If you build it, they will come").

Applied to your life, it goes like this: "Create the space. Something will come in."

Remember, right now I'm not asking you to *do* anything. I just want you to start making space for exercise and health, maybe just in your mind. Be open to it. Hang out with the possibility. Then watch what happens to that space when you least expect it.

Something will fill it.

And if you're already exercising or live a very active life, list some ways you could up the ante. Maybe that aerobics class you take twice a week is getting ho-hum. Or that thirty minutes you've been doing on the treadmill is starting to feel like sleepwalking. How about some interval training? A 5K race? The kickboxing class you've been hearing about? What would take you to the next level? Think about it.

3. Take a fresh sheet in your journal—actually, you might want to reserve a few pages for this one.   We're going to call it your "to-do" list, and we'll be talking more about how it fits into the program later on. For now, here's what I want you to do: *Make a list of actions or tasks that you've been putting off that would make a difference to you if you completed them.* They can be small, easy actions, like returning a phone call or straightening up a closet, or they can be significant, like clearing up a misunderstanding with a friend or parent that's been festering between the two of you for a long time. Don't get stuck on the meaning of the phrase "making a difference." (And remember, don't get sucked into paying too much attention to those little voices in your head that I warned you about, the ones that are asking what all this has to do with weight loss. Just trust me on this one for now.) To get a place on the list, an action doesn't have to be something gigantic—like getting engaged or divorced or going back to school—but it *could* be. Sometimes just getting a phone bill paid or clearing out that old pile of Sunday newspapers near the bed creates a little whisper of mental fresh air that comes from finally doing something you've been putting off. There's no right way to make your list. Just do it. You'll read more about the to-do list in the next chapter, where you'll find a lot more detailed information on how to make this exercise really work for you. It's a big part of the program, so don't neglect it.

4. Take an inventory of your kitchen. Throw out some things that you *know* don't need to be there during the next eight weeks. Look ahead at the food lists in Chapter 5 and see if there are some things you might want to stock up on. At this point in the game, you may not be clear about which foods to keep and which ones to toss. (I'm going to steadfastly refuse to use the terms "allowed" and "forbidden" when it comes to food. Sorry!) But I'll bet you have some ideas. Go with your instincts for now. During the course of the program you'll undoubtedly be relearning (and un-learning) some of your most treasured concepts about what constitutes healthy eating, but for now, let's go with the obvious: potato chips and Twinkies, for example, aren't going to make the cut. Look for foods that you have your own personal battles with, foods that trigger eating binges, foods you are most likely to overeat.

If you live in a house with other people, such as a roommate, kids or a spouse, this exercise can be tricky, since it's *you* that's doing the Shape Up program, not everyone in the house, and you're undoubtedly going to meet with some resistance if you start acting like the food police and throwing out everyone else's favorite snacks. One technique that has worked for a lot of people who've done the program is to appropriate a separate section of the cupboard for yourself. Maybe you can commandeer one cabinet or even one section of the refrigerator—at least for now—and earmark it just for you.

5. Find a quiet time when you won't be disturbed, sit in a pleasant and peaceful place and answer the following questions. Really take your time with them. You may want to answer some right away and ponder others at your leisure. It's not necessary to finish these four short lists before beginning the program, though I'd suggest you give it a try with the understanding that you may want to come back during the next eight weeks and edit, add to or modify your answers in some way.

The answers to the questions are yours alone. Remember that there are absolutely no right or wrong answers. Be truthful and you will get much more out of the process.

• **Make a list of the three things you most like about your body.** *(Hint: Don't say "nothing." That's not allowed. It can be anything, from your* *skin, to your fingernails, to your smile, to the shape of a particular body part. If you honestly can't think of one thing, make something up.)*

- Make a list of the three things you most dislike about your body. (*No more than three!*)

- Make a list of three things you could do right now that would make a difference today. *(Hint: These things could be as simple as refusing dessert just for tonight or cutting portions in half for just one meal. And here's a note to your inner voice: Don't invalidate whatever you come up with by saying "Well, that wouldn't make that much of a difference." That's not what's important here. What's important here is that you list something—some tangible action—that would be a step, no matter how small, in the direction you want to go. We'll worry about how big or important it's going to turn out to be later.)*

- Make a list of three things that you are giving up by not being fitter and having a body you can be happy in. What is it costing you? (*If you're really ambitious and want some extra credit, try tackling this one as well: What do you gain by keeping things the way they are? What's the hidden payoff?*)

FOOD

"Are bananas good?"

"Is fruit juice bad?"

"Is it OK to eat bagels?"

I personally try to avoid one word answers to those questions, not because I want to frustrate people, but because I want them to understand that with few exceptions (I'll mention some of those in a minute) most foods are like vacation resorts: they have their good points and they have their bad. If you like skiing and don't mind snow, Aspen is the place to be, but if you're a beach person, it's your idea of purgatory. By being clear about what your priorities and needs are, you can look at a food and decide whether *on balance* it's something you want to include on a regular basis, something you should limit or something you should avoid as much as possible.

Take orange juice, for example. It's got folic acid, which is good. But it's also high in sugar and low in fiber, both of which are *not* good. If you're trying to sell orange juice to people, you emphasize the folic acid content. But on balance, in my opinion, the plus of the folic acid doesn't outweigh the high amount of sugar and the complete absence of fiber. For weight control, the decision is clear: Forget the juice and eat the orange. There are much better ways to get folic acid, and the high sugar content and lack of fiber in the juice make eating the whole fruit a far better choice.

Bagels are an even easier call. They're nothing more than highly processed flour which converts to sugar very quickly in the body. The processing removes most of the nutrients and practically all of the fiber, leaving you with a high-calorie, low-nutrient, fiberless junk food. And the proponents of the food pyramid want to convince you it's a health food!

If giving up bagels represents a real challenge for you, you're not alone. There is, however, a solution. Simply minimize the damage by not letting it be the centerpiece of your breakfast. Instead, try hollowing it out and putting in some nut butter, like almond butter or peanut butter; then eat it with a small apple. Or try something unusual, like topping it with a couple of slices of turkey. Protein (in the turkey), fat (in the almond butter) and fiber (in the apple) all slow down the body's sugar response to the bagel and help balance the meal. The practical result? Better energy levels for longer periods of time.

As an added benefit, many people notice that when they add some fat, protein or fiber to the morning meal, they experience a remarkable decrease in mid-morning cravings. Those cravings are almost always the result of a blood sugar roller coaster put in motion by a typical high-car-bohydrate, low-fiber breakfast, a breakfast which often has bread as the centerpiece of the meal.

Some foods, however, have little ambiguity about them and land firmly in the "avoid at all costs" list. Margarine is a good example. This man-made food was engineered in response to the fat-phobic environment so preva-lent in the 1980s (and still hanging on for dear life). The only problem was that the "cure" turned out to be worse than the "disease." Margarine con-tains a class of fats called trans-fatty acids, mutated, unnatural fats that sci-entists are finding cause far more damage than the more natural saturated fat in the butter it's meant to replace. People in the know are strongly rec-ommending that you eliminate margarine altogether. I couldn't agree more. Reasonable amounts of pure, good quality butter can easily be worked into a well-constructed diet, and the butter won't do any of the damage that the trans-fats in margarine will do, and may even do you some good.

Some foods have so many great qualities that they can be almost uni-versally recommended. But even some of these may have a property that you may want to know about, which may temper how much you use it. Let's take the lowly brussels sprout. Hard to find anything wrong with it. Green vegetable, loaded with vitamins, nutrients, fiber. And here's some-thing else that's great about it that you may not have known: Brussels sprouts contain something that help activate phase 2 detoxification path-ways in the liver. What a deal, right?

But if you have a sluggish thyroid, you may want to modify your intake of brussels sprouts. Brussels sprouts, as a member of the cruciferous fam-ily (which also includes broccoli), may have a slightly slowing effect on the thyroid in susceptible people. Same with tomatoes and eggplants. Great foods, unless you have gout. The take-home point is this: Even the best foods in the world may not always be right for some people under some circumstances.

With the understanding that individual differences—such as food sen-sitivities, special conditions and personal preferences—always need to be honored, we can still make some general rules.

• High-sugar foods tend invariably to lead to sluggishness and cravings after the initial sugar buzz wears off. And they tend to foster cravings.

- Protein, on the other hand, frequently produces feeling of mental energy., and also tends to keep us less hungry.
- High-fiber foods have many health benefits; they also slow the absorption of other foods, creating a more even energy level for a longer period of time. (The ultimate high-fiber food is beans, which have only one real disadvantage, and this can easily be remedied with a little Bean-O.)

Almost any food can be incorporated into the diet if you're doing everything else right. The trick is to look at the whole picture. If you're eating enough protein, vegetables, omega-3 fats and fiber, you can probably sneak in a Twinkie without doing much damage. But if it's Twinkies and McDonald's all day long, well, that's a very different story.

Language can be a great aid in this. I encourage people to stop thinking of foods as good or bad. Think of food as a kind of purchase, and then ask yourself if it's a good value. If there are both positives and negatives, does one outweigh the other? Is this a food that supports your goal? By asking these kinds of questions you empower yourself with information; you take charge of your own diet instead of blindly following the recommendations of others.

Sure, it's harder this way. Sure, we wish the world were simpler. But in the long run going beyond just good and bad will give you infinitely greater satisfaction.

And much better results.

The Food Lists: What Can I Eat?

> To attain knowledge, add things every day.
> To attain wisdom, remove things every day.
>
> —*LAO TSU*

Eavesdrop on enough conversations among dieters and certain patterns begin to emerge. Themes reveal themselves, and like the plot lines of soap operas, they recycle with predictable regularity. Bring up any new diet in conversation, and undoubtedly the first question you'll be asked is the same question I get asked the most on-line, at seminars, by callers to my radio show and in my private practice. It's probably one you yourself have undoubtedly asked at one point or another:

"What can I eat?"

This is usually followed by some variation on "How much?" and "How often?"

Well, I don't blame you for wanting to know. When you're making your way through the jungles of the diet wars, you tend to want a map. And there is no shortage of diet gurus willing to give you theirs, the one and only "right" one.

But there are both pros and cons to following someone's rigid program.

The main pro is that a formal diet plan gives you *structure*. It takes away uncertainty and replaces it with a prescription. It acts in loco parentis: You get very specific rules about what *foods* (or *classes* of foods) you must never eat (*Dr. Atkins's New Diet Revolution, The Pritikin Program*), or what *combinations* of foods you must (or must not) eat (*Somersizing, The Zone*), or what *time of day* you may eat them (*Fit for Life*) or what *amounts* are acceptable (Weight Watchers, or virtually any guide to low-calorie eating).

Any women's magazine with a menu plan that begins with

Breakfast:
1/2 grapefruit
1 slice whole wheat toast
1 tablespoon jam

is catering to that need for certainty and structure. You've all seen these food plans. You've probably even tried a few. This paint-by-numbers"approach promises maximum results with minimum effort and is almost always accompanied by inspirational testimonies of the "look how it worked for me" variety. They're tempting indeed. What could be easier?

I understand the appeal of such programs. And I'm not saying they don't work—for some people, some of the time. But herein lies the rub: People don't stay with them.

To begin with, some of these styles of eating are so different from what you're used to that they contain the seeds of their own defeat. Sure, you can tell a person who has eaten most of her meals at McDonald's for the past five years to go on a macrobiotic diet of fruit and rice, but how long is she going to last on that? Sure, you can tell a meat-and-potatoes gal to cut out all carbs, but is that realistic? Or you can tell her to measure and weigh each portion, or to count calories obsessively, or fat grams, or carbohydrate content, but can you ask her to live that way forever? Especially since she doesn't want to?

These programs never take into account individual differences in metabolism, digestion, personal style, food allergies, appetite, preferences, or any of the other individual factors that I've mentioned in this book. They violate the number one rule of social work, which is: "Meet the client where she lives." These programs give a hungry woman a fish, but they don't show her how to use a fishing pole. They impose a structure *on* you rather than teaching you how to develop your own. How much better would it be to work with and honor your own individuality? And use that individuality to evolve and develop an eating program that works for *you*, and that you can live with forever?

The beauty of the Shape Up program is that you can begin it from wherever you are, *right now*. You start at *your* own starting point, which is your current way of eating. And over the course of the eight weeks, you're going to begin to learn how foods affect *you*; which ones contribute to your well-being, which ones increase your energy, which ones make you feel bloated and tired and which ones keep you from losing weight. And those may not be the exact same foods that make your neighbor (or me) feel good (or bad).

I'm going to ask you to experiment, with my structured guidance, and see what happens when you eliminate or reduce certain foods. I'm going to discourage you from thinking of foods in simplistic terms like "good" and "bad," and encourage you instead to think in terms of what results they produce. Not just the result of weight loss, though that's certainly one that you'll experience, but the result of vibrant good health, improved mood and energy and an increased sense of personal power.

Now, the downside of my approach is that it doesn't always give you clear-cut rules to follow. But that only shows up as a downside because of our desperate need for clear-cut maps and because following a map is always easier than developing our own powerful sense of direction. I'm going to help you discover that powerful sense of self-determination and direction, but it's going to wind up being *your* sense of direction, for *your* life, for the body *you* want and deserve. It's not going to be one I've imposed on you.

Because in the end, the Shape Up program is about the one thing you can't get from meal plans, inflexible rules or authoritarian diets.

It's about personal power.

And that's something that you get to keep for the rest of your life.

How to Use the Food Lists

Designing your personal eating program for weight loss and health on the Shape Up plan couldn't be easier. There are two lists, an "A" list and a "B" list. The idea is to begin choosing foods from the "A" list as often as possible and to begin *reducing* foods on the "B" list as much as possible. It's as simple as that. (There's a third group, the "C" list, which I'll discuss later.)

In the early days of Shape Up, foods were divided into two basic categories: "Foods to Add" and "Foods to Avoid." I changed the headings because it left some people with the impression that they could *never* eat anything on the "Foods to Avoid" list. But Shape Up is about designing a strategy that works for *you*. There will be some people for whom "B" list foods work on occasion and some people for whom they just don't work at all. Here's the truth: If you were left on a desert island for a year, you would survive and thrive if the only foods available to you were those on the "A" list. You don't *need* the foods on the "B" list—they would keep you just barely alive on that mythical desert island and even then only if they were fortified with enough synthetic vitamins and trace amounts of protein and fat to keep you from croaking. Does this mean you can never eat them? No, of course not. And how *much* you eat them will be up to you. But to the extent that you can make the shift over to the "A" side, you will see results with your weight and your health.

How completely do you have to make that shift? Well, that's a very individual thing, which we'll discuss in even more detail in Chapter 18 ("It's a War Out There"). Some people have a metabolism that is fairly forgiving, and may not require strict adherence to the "A" list at all times. Others will need to be stricter to get the results they want and will need to really limit their ventures into "B" territory to just once in a while. Some people, when they begin really making the shift and seeing results, will find that their desire for the foods on the "B" list has really diminished and may choose to live almost exclusively on the "A" list. This is where the power of the Shape Up program lies, because it is based on the concept of biochemical individuality and psychological uniqueness. You get to try things out and see what works for *you*.

Another thing you need to know about the Shape Up eating guidelines is the principle of "add before you subtract." You can't tear up the foundation of a house all at once, and it's the same thing with an eating style. That's why the Shape Up program focuses first on *adding* foods to your current diet. The foods on the "A" list provide immediate health benefits and you should add as many of them as you can to your daily diet. The foods on the "B" list get in the way of weight loss and contribute next to nothing to your health. Don't worry if your favorite foods are on the "B" list. For right now, focus on adding what's on the "A" list. There's time to reduce the "B" list foods as we get a little further along.

"A" List

- **Vegetables.** These are the best things to add to your diet, and you can add them in unlimited amounts. Think in terms of color: Try to add every color to your shopping basket—red, orange, white and especially green. Vegetables provide fiber, nutrients, antioxidants, phytochemicals and enzymes in a low-calorie package, all of which help you lose weight and gain health. Following is a partial list of vegetables to choose from. You can prepare them with olive oil or a little fresh creamy butter, and with as many seasonings as you like (herbs and spices that are particularly recommended are listed later in this section).

Spinach	Alfalfa sprouts
Broccoli	Collard Greens
Cauliflower	Cucumbers
Kale	Mushrooms
Snow peas	Onions
Carrots	Peppers (all colors)
Beets	Brussels Sprouts
Squash	Cabbage
Green beans	Celery
Asparagus	Eggplant
Turnips	Leeks
Fresh corn	Okra
on the cob	Parsnips
Peas	Tomatoes

- **Water.** Involved in every cellular process, water is the best weight-loss drink in the world. Forget the "eight glasses a day" recommendation and drink as much as you can, as often as you'd like. (Fruit juice and soda are not substitutes, and coffee definitely doesn't count because, among other things, it's a diuretic.) You should make every effort to get pure bottled or filtered water.

- **Fish.** In general, the more the better. If you can eat it several times a week that's great. One of the greatest health foods in the world is a can of sardines—and it's cheap, too! Following is a partial list of seafood from which to choose:

Tuna	Bluefish
Mackerel	Flounder
Whitefish	Yellowtail
Salmon	Mahi mahi
Grouper	Scallops
Sardines	Shrimp

- **Eggs.** Eggs are one of nature's most perfect foods. They contain everything needed to support life. Eggs have been given a terrible rap in the popular press over the last decade and, as you'll find out in the later sections of this book, a very unfair one. Eat them and enjoy them, and this includes the yolks, which are a superb source of vitamin A and of phosphatidylcholine. Phosphatidylcholine is needed to form lecithin, which helps prevent cholesterol from being oxidized,and is also a superb nutrient for liver health. Eggs also contain lutein and zeaxanthin, powerful carotenoids that are critical in protecting the eye against macular degeneration. Dr. Fred Pescatore, author of *Feed Your Kids Right,* says, "If you buy one food that's organic, make it eggs." Organic eggs from free-range chickens are far more likely to contain a healthful amount of beneficial omega-3 fats, and some eggs now come with an omega-3 guarantee on the box. Buy them!

- **Whey protein powder.** This is one of the most absorbable and bioavailable sources of protein on the planet, and it's inexpensive and versatile. Whey protein is also very immuno-protective and causes the body to make more of one of its most critically important antioxidants, glutathione. It's great in shakes and can also be mixed with oatmeal. Shakes—especially made with whey protein—are a great way to get protein when you're crunched for time and can't sit down and eat. We're going to eventually try for protein at every meal, so be creative.

- **Meat.** There is no inherent problem with eating meat, but the meat that is commonly available in supermarkets is unfortunately also a source of a lot of things we don't want, such as antibiotics and toxins. To get all the benefits of meat while minimizing the problems, you need to do some careful shopping. Veal and lamb are good choices, as are the leanest cuts of Angus beef and anything that is organically grown. The cuts from muscles that work hard are coarser in texture but have much less fat—examples are rump, eye round, flank steak and brisket. Whenever possible, try to get meat that is lean antibiotic and steroid-free. And don't rule out lean, trimmed, tender meats such as pork tenderloin and roast.

• **Poultry.** Free-range, antibiotic-free poultry is really worth the extra money if you can manage it

• **Salads.** The addition of a salad a day, preferably before a meal, can do wonders for appetite management, not to mention the fiber, nutrients, phytochemicals and antioxidants you'll be getting. Garnish with some nuts (see next item). By the way, this is also a great way to get some raw foods into your diet (see "A Word About Preparation Methods")

• **Nuts.** Nuts can be a great source of protein, essential fatty acids and minerals. I'm not suggesting you sit and munch on handfuls of peanuts (which aren't nuts, anyway, but legumes), but I *am* suggesting you include nuts in your diet on a regular basis. About a quarter or a cup is a good starting point for a portion. Think P-A-W for pecans, almonds and walnuts, which have the best mixture of good fats and minerals, though raw cashews, filberts, macadamia nuts and Brazil nuts are fine too. And don't be afraid of a tablespoon of delicious, preferably organic, nut butters like almond, cashew or even peanut smeared on a stick of celery or half an apple. Try it—it's delicious.

→ With nuts, as with many foods, you have to be aware of your personal idiosyncratic reaction. Great as they may be, nuts are also subject to mold and rancidity, a definite problem for many people, especially those with yeast (candida). And some people are allergic. You can increase the odds of getting all the benefits by getting fresh, raw nuts and soaking them in water overnight, which makes them far more digestible. Sally Fallon, author of *Nourishing Traditions,* recommends draining them after an overnight soak and then toasting them in the oven on a baking sheet.

• **Fruit (especially berries).** Aim for up to two fruits a day, and choose from the lower-sugar kind, like grapefruits, plums, apricots, apples and pears, and especially blueberries, raspberries and strawberries.

They will give you healthful benefits without much of a problem from a weight loss standpoint. This is not an "unlimited" item, though, because many fruits are high in sugar and too much of them can create a scenario in your body that isn't conducive to weight loss. Ripe bananas, which are a staple of the low-fat diet programs and which many people devour like candy, are a high-sugar item—especially when eaten alone. Use with discretion, or eat them when they are firm.

• **Olive oil.** A couple of tablespoonfuls a day, preferably of the extra virgin, cold-pressed variety, is a very good idea. It's even better if it's not heated (i.e., used on salads or vegetables), but it is the preferred oil for cooking as well as eating.

• **Other good fats.** Most people who have been following the low-fat diet dogma are woefully underconsuming good fats. Paradoxically, some fats (like the omega-3 fats found in fish and flaxseed, and GLA, a particular omega-6 fat found in evening primrose oil) can actually help you *lose* body fat. These fatty acids "sit" on the cell membrane and act as a cheerleader, encouraging other fats to get into the cell where they can be burned for fuel. Fat, incidentally, has virtually no effect on insulin levels. Hopefully you're learning in this book why the wholesale avoidance of fats was a very, very bad idea in the first place. The trick is to correct it by eating the right ones. Following is a partial list of fats—or foods that contain them—that you can begin including in your diet:

> Flaxseed oil (but don't cook with it)
> Flaxseed meal
> Avocados
> Nuts
> Nut butters
> Sesame tahini
> Seeds
> Coconut
> Coconut oil
> Butter (in reasonable amounts)
> And of course the fats found in cold-water fish,
>   like salmon, tuna, mackerel and sardines

• **Spices and herbs.** Cinnamon, turmeric, ginger, any green leafy herbs and plants in the mint family (for example, rosemary, basil, mint, peppermint, spearmint, thyme and lemon balm), garlic (in all its forms), cayenne pepper, cloves, parsley, cumin seed. Most are loaded with antioxidants, and all have health-giving properties. Use liberally and often.

• **Green tea.** Black tea has nearly as much of the antioxidant power as green tea, so you could use that as well.

• **Fresh-squeezed vegetable juices.**

The Importance of the Glycemic Index

You may be aware that there has been a great deal of discussion among nutritionists and in the media about the "glycemic index" of food. Briefly, the glycemic index is a measure of how quickly a specific food raises your blood sugar. Knowing how fast a food you eat breaks down into sugar can be very important in weight management. And that's where knowing the glycemic index can be helpful. Foods with a high glycemic index raise blood sugar quickly; those with a low glycemic index do not.

When blood sugar goes up, the pancreas responds with a shot of the hormone insulin. Insulin is a storage hormone—one of its jobs is to escort the sugar from the blood into the cells, thus bringing blood sugar levels back down to normal. When you constantly eat meals that are extremely high glycemic, you're constantly raising both blood sugar levels and insulin levels and setting yourself up for the blood sugar roller coaster ride that inevitably leads to cravings, mood swings and huge shifts in energy. The body doesn't burn fat in the presence of high levels of insulin. Keeping insulin levels from being chronically elevated is probably one of the best overall weight loss strategies you can adapt (not to mention that it is good for your health in general and at the top of the list of anti-aging strategies).

There are a few things to keep in mind about the glycemic index:
• Remember that the glycemic index applies only to foods eaten alone. When you mix stuff together, it's like mixing paint of different colors—the result is something different than any of the individual

ingredients. Adding nut butters to a piece of fruit or turkey to a high-glycemic rice cake brings down the glycemic load of the meal .

- Sometimes the version of a food makes a big difference. For example, sweet potatoes and regular white potatoes are quite different; instant oatmeal and real, steel-cut, slow-cooking oatmeal are very different; and ripe bananas and hard bananas are somewhat different. An apple with its chewy fiber enters into the system a lot slower then that same apple made into apple juice.

- There are two different versions of the glycemic index floating around—one uses pure glucose as the standard (100) the other assigns 100 to white bread and rates everything proportionally from there (resulting in some foods having ratings as high as 164). The important thing to know is which foods are relatively low, which are relatively high and which are medium. And remember that the glycemic index is not the *whole* picture when it comes to either health or insulin production, just a part of it.

Finally, the glycemic index, while important, isn't the only thing you need to pay attention to when choosing foods. A food can be low-glycemic and still be junk, while some higher-glycemic foods—watermelon, for example—are good for you. And once in a while, a food may have a low glycemic index but can still impact health in a negative way. Fructose, for example, is often touted as a "good" sugar because it has a low glycemic index, but it happens to raise triglycerides in the blood more than any other sugar and has a greater tendency to be converted to fat. And there are some foods that have a strong insulin-raising effect even though they don't have a high glycemic index—sucrose, for example.

The moral of the story: By all means pay attention to the glycemic index, and especially to sugar in all its forms, but don't use it as a substitute for thinking about what you're eating. Most foods that raise blood sugar quickly are commercial breads, cereals, pastas, crackers, snack foods, and desserts. Some vegetables, such as carrots and beets, have a high glycemic index, and for that reason they have wound up on some diet plan "hit lists." I don't agree with this approach. The benefits of these foods far outweigh the minor detail of their high-glycemic index. I also agree with diabetes expert and nutritional researcher C. Leigh Broadhurst that "no one ever became diabetic by eating peas and carrots.

While it's true that a few vegetables have a relatively high sugar content, they come in such a rich package of nutrients that there is no reason to avoid them. Let's choose our battles carefully. There are far more important foods to take off the menu. Protein, good fat, tons of vegetables, some fruit, and lots of fiber—that's the core of the Shape Up program. Dump the commercial breads, pastas, cereals, cakes, snack foods, and desserts, and you won't have to worry about which vegetables are OK.

"B" List

- **Commercial breads.** Most of these have had all the good stuff processed out, even though many manufacturers attempt to make them look like warm and fuzzy health foods. Flour by definition is pulverized and defiberized grain and rarely has anything of benefit left in it. Most of the vitamins are lost in the processing. The manufacturer then throws a few paltry ones back in (hence the term "enriched"), which is rather like robbing the bank and leaving the tellers money for coffee. The only *possible* exception to the rule would be breads that are genuinely made with whole grains, but these are much harder to find than you would think and definitely don't include most supermarket imposters. Get into the habit of reading the label for ingredients. Occasionally you will come across some breads that are actually made without flour—the ingredients will list, for example, whole grain rye, yeast, water and salt, or seven different whole grains. (One of the best, though it's an acquired taste, is Ezekiel bread.) In addition, most breads are high-glycemic and provoke an insulin response that you don't want. For that reason, I think it's a good idea to really limit them, at least for a while, and see how you feel. Breads are also very easy to overeat.

→Be aware that many people have a food sensitivity to gliadin, a fraction of gluten which is found mainly in wheat but also in many other grains. This sensitivity may not be a full-blown allergy, but it can show up as symptoms ranging from water retention and bloating to headaches, weight gain and "brain fog." More people than you might imagine have this sensitivity, and if you are one of them, any grain that contains gluten, and definitely any wheat product, is going to be a problem for you. This includes couscous (which is tiny pasta) and tabouli (which is cracked wheat). Many people are amazed at how good they feel when they remove wheat from their diet. You may not be one of them, but it's definitely worth finding out if you are. If you're not ready to go all the way and eliminate wheat for a period of time, you might want to experiment by seriously reducing your consumption, or by trying gluten-free grains. Some "halfway house" alternatives that are a big improvement over commercial wheat products include polenta or cornbread, provided you make it with a whole grain cornmeal (like Arrowhead Mills). Remember, though, that these are still high-carb, high-calorie items that should come with a "handle with care" label.

- **Bagels.** Contrary to popular belief, these are anything but a health food. They contain the worst of everything that's wrong with bread, calorie-wise they cost a pretty penny. If you must indulge, scoop out the doughy, yeasty middle part and eat the crust, preferably with some nut butter, turkey, or salmon. Better yet, leave them alone.

- **Commercial pastas.** Virtually everything true of breads (above) is also true of pasta. In addition, the portions we commonly consume of this food are simply outrageous. If you're not ready to give it up completely, use it as a small side dish and limit it as much as possible. Load it up with vegetables, add some protein and a little olive oil. Don't make it a main dish, and don't consume it often.

- **Cakes and pies.** This category also includes desserts, doughnuts, and any other packaged little cakes or cupcakes.

- **Commercial cereals.** Sadly, this includes virtually everything on the supermarket shelf that comes in a box with a cute little picture on it. The good news is that it doesn't include oatmeal, buckwheat groats (kasha), and whole grain grits. These are good starches. The same caveats about breads apply here, though—don't overconsume.

- **Packaged snack foods.** Chips, candy bars, crackers, and yes, pretzels too.

- **Refined vegetable oils.** This is one of the worst items on the list. Don't eat them or cook with them. I'm talking about virtually every common supermarket oil *including* canola, which is loaded with toxins and has been falsely marketed as healthy because it contains some omega-3 fats (however, that very fact makes it a bad choice for cooking). If you can find cold-pressed, organic canola oil that would be OK, but even then I wouldn't heat it to high temperatures. Avoid like the plague refined corn oil, sunflower oil, safflower oil, soy oil and other supermarket fare. If you really need these oils, it is truly worth making the trip to the health food store and spending the extra money for cold-pressed, unrefined virgin oils. Remember that even the best vegetable oils are still mostly omega-6's and heavy reliance on them exacerbates the imbalance between the 6's that we overconsume and the 3's that we underconsume. Experiment with alternative sources like flaxseed, sesame, pistachio, walnut, hazelnut and grapeseed. Get the best quality you can find and mix and match your fats. Use extra-virgin (cold-pressed) olive oil whenever possible. Reasonable amounts of fresh butter are fine, and for cooking, peanut and coconut oil, or *real* lard (not Crisco!).

- **Margarine.** A trans-fatty acid orgy, one of the stupidest mistakes ever made by the food industry. It's a disgrace that some of the establishment groups actually endorsed this stuff as "heart healthy." Go back to butter.

- **Sugar.** This may be the hardest to give up (you may have to do it gradually), but to the extent that you can do it, you will experience profound and dramatic results in both weight loss and general health. Remember, table sugar is only the most obvious form; there are about nineteen other disguises in which it sneaks into our food. The result: We manage to ingest about 135 pounds of sugar per person per year. We'll be talking a lot more about sugar later in this book.

- **Sodas.** A neat little package of sugar, calories, chemicals, and caffeine, and a calcium robber if there ever was one. Not one good thing about it, unless you're comparing it to heroin.

- **Diet sodas.** The evidence is overwhelming that they don't help you lose weight at all, and the evidence is compelling that they do you far more harm than good.
- **Fruit juice.** This is a pure sugar hit, and definitely not a health food. It has little of the good stuff in the fruit, and no fiber to slow the

effect on blood sugar and insulin levels. If you do have a blender like Vita Mix or a juicer, and you make your own, I still recommend that you make a mix using mostly vegetables and a smaller amount of fruit. The only exception to the store-bought fruit juice rule would be unsweetened cranberry juice, which is hard to find, very tart, and rather expensive. However, it provides a lot of digestive enzymes and when diluted with water makes a nice morning drink.

"Good" Fats and "Bad" Fats

If you're still confused about the difference between "good" fats and "bad" fats and are wondering why we even need fats in our diets if we're trying to lose weight, the simple answer is this: Your body creates some very important substances—called eicosanoids, or prostaglandins—out of fats. It also uses fats to build important hormones, and to build the cell walls, and to transport vitamins like A, D, and E. So think of fats as bricks that a contractor would use for building sections of your house. The better the bricks, the stronger the building. If there are only broken or damaged bricks around, the contractor *will* use them (since the house has to be built), but the house won't be as strong and eventually there will be problems.

Good fats are basically the naturally occurring, traditional fats that haven't been damaged by high heat, refining, processing or other man-made tampering like partial hydrogenation. The very best of these are found in fish, nuts, avocados, seeds and even, believe it or not, fresh creamy butter. Animal fats have a bad reputation, but many of us believe it is not animal fats per se that are bad but the combination of *high* consumption of fats from toxic animals coupled with *low* consumption of fiber and vegetables, the very combination that is usually seen in every study that shows an association between animal products and various diseases. Because of horrible factory farming methods, and the widespread use of antibiotics and steroids, animal fats from non–organically raised, non–free range animals should probably be used with prudence. One of the worst of the bad fats is margarine, as are the fats found in anything that's fried. And if you see "partially hydrogenated" anything on the label, run like the dickens.

Refined vegetable oils like you find in the average supermarket are definitely on my personal hit list for bad fats. They oxidize easily (think of a sliced apple left out in the open air) and have been processed with high heat and chemicals, which further damages them. They have a nice long shelf life, but the only people who benefit from that are the manufacturers—rodents won't even touch the stuff, which makes it good from a business point of view, horrible from the point of view of your body. Extra virgin, cold-pressed olive oil, however, is a good fat.

Unfortunately, some of the best fats, like flaxseed oil, and fish oils, can't be used for cooking. The very thing that makes them so good for you also makes them unstable, and they respond badly to high heat. If you must cook with high heat, you're better off with something like peanut oil, coconut oil, or even real lard (*not* the vegetable shortening sold in supermarkets). These are far more stable. Of course, not cooking with very high heat would be the best of all.

Good fats come from fish, avocados, nuts, seeds, extra virgin, cold-pressed olive oil, coconut, butter and other traditional foods. Use them in reasonable amounts and they will help you stay healthy. Remember the Weston Price studies of fourteen vibrantly healthy native societies that I talked about in Chapter 2? It's worth noting that not one of them was on a low-fat diet.

"C" List

You may be wondering what happened to the foods that aren't on either the "A" or the "B" list. Remember that one other list I told you we'd be talking about? Well, here it is, and those missing foods are on it. Here's why: There are a number of foods that are very problematic for some people, while others seem to be able to do fine with them. I've put these foods on a third short list, the "C" list. My suggestion is that you monitor your reaction to them very carefully and decide whether or not they fit into your strategy at all, and if so, to what extent.

- **Starches.** This is not an "all you can eat" category. All starches are not bad, contrary to some misinterpretations in the media, but an awful lot of them are junk as well as being major saboteurs of weight loss. And, unfortunately, if fat loss is a goal, you will probably have to choose them very carefully and limit the portion sizes. However, that said, there *is* a short list of starches that are great health foods. My favorites are sweet potatoes (or yams), oatmeal (not the instant kind, but the steel-cut, slow-cooking type), and almost all lentils and beans. As mentioned earlier, whole grain grits and buckwheat groats (kasha) are acceptable as well. Rice has a low allergen potential (unlike many other grains) but is a high-starch food that can easily sabotage weight loss. If you are careful about the size of your portions there's no reason you can't include these in your plan. Many people find that one starch a day is a good place to begin while they figure out their best strategy.

• **Milk.** I do not believe supermarket milk is a good food for adults or children, for reasons that would take us too far afield but have been well documented elsewhere. Homogenization changes the nature of the fat, pasteurization destroys the enzymes, the protein in milk (casein) is a major allergen, most of the world is lactose intolerant, and dairy is extremely mucus-forming for a large segment of the population. The wholesale use of bovine growth hormone to increase milk production troubles me greatly. Although I know some conscientious dairy farmers who have assured me that government inspections for antibiotics in the milk are very thorough (cows are injected with antibiotics to deal with the mastitis brought on by factory farming methods and the artificially increased milk production brought on by rBGH), critics have made a compelling case for why we should not be so sanguine. I have no objection to raw, certified milk (if you can find it), organic milk, or milk from a small family farm, but in my opinion modern processing has taken what once might have been a very healthy food (for some, anyway) and turned it into something that it is very difficult to recommend for anyone. In fairness, some people do seem to do OK with milk, but enough people have told me that their lives have changed (and their weight loss plateaus ended) when they eliminated dairy (and/or wheat) for me to recommend that you at least consider removing it for a while to see if it makes a difference.

• **Other dairy.** Though I tend not to recommend dairy for all people, there are some people who tolerate it better than others. For those people, cottage cheese and other soft cheeses, like feta and farmer, can be treated as "A" list foods. Goat cheese is superb. Even hard cheeses for those who tolerate them, are fine on occasion, particularly Swiss, which, by the way, is a far better source of calcium than milk. If you're buying hard cheeses, look for those made from raw milk. If you even suspect a yeast problem, avoid the fermented kind, like blue cheese and Roquefort. Yogurt is fine as long as it's *not* the no-fat kind, which is loaded with sugar, and as long as it has real live cultures. If you can find them, the sheep's milk and goat's milk varieties of yogurt are great tasting and extremely nutritious.

• **Coffee.** Frankly, I'm still on the fence on this one. Unquestionably, coffee stresses the adrenals, which are the glands responsible for stress hormones. It releases sugar into the bloodstream, thus stimulating an insulin response, and has been known to sabotage weight loss efforts if for no other reason than its association with foods that do. If you are always getting your energy from stimulants like caffeine, it is that much more difficult to really get to understand the effect your food (and your lifestyle) is having on you. You never know if your food is producing energy and alertness or if it's producing tiredness and fatigue—you're masking the effects of both your lifestyle (sleep habits, stress responses) and your eating style with a powerful stimulant. And that just might be keeping you from valuable knowledge about which foods work for you and which ones don't.

→ Coffee also increases urinary secretion of minerals like magnesium, potassium, and sodium, and uses up a fair amount of vitamin B-1. And it can raise blood pressure and interfere with sleep. In addition, the plant itself is a repository of toxins and pesticides, by some counts more than 200 of them.

On the other hand, it's a hard thing to give up, and it affects some people much more than others. That said, there are things you can do to minimize the negatives if you're not ready to dump it entirely. First is to buy organic. Second is to buy fresh beans, keep them in an airtight container and grind them right before you use them (reducing or preventing rancidity). And finally, use brown (unbleached) filters, since then at least you won't be adding bleach to the mix.

The number of additional junk calories taken in daily by people consuming designer triple soy mochaccinos or whatever the caffeine-sugar-dairy-laden *latte du jour* happens to be is a major contributor to the growing waistline of America. But if you enjoy it as a special treat once in a while, and you don't live on the stuff, you should be fine.

• **Alcohol.** If ever there was a substance that perfectly illustrated the metaphor "double-edged sword," alcohol is surely it. On the one hand, numerous studies have shown that moderate—let me emphasize the word moderate—drinkers live longer and have less heart disease. Red wine, for example, contains a number of health-promoting bioflavonoids, such as resveratrol, quercetin and rutin. And there is mounting evidence that it's not just the compounds in the wine—

there is something about the alcohol *per se* that may be helpful in getting those bioflavonoids in the wine into our systems. In addition, the relaxing experience created by moderate alcohol drinking probably reduces levels of the stress hormone cortisol, which, when elevated, leads to a lot of nasty stuff, including abdominal weight gain.

Critics say there is nothing in wine that you couldn't get just as well from grapes and other fruits and vegetables ('cept, of course, the relaxing and unwinding experience). But this too is a double-edged sword. I've seen more people than I can count unwind with some alcohol and before you know it consume *waaay* more food than they ever intended to, and rarely of the kind that's going to keep them on track. Casually sipping a drink—wine or otherwise—while preparing dinner or during cocktail hour has been the undoing of more than one person trying to reshape his or her body. Alcohol has a way of relaxing not only *social* inhibitions, but *eating* inhibitions as well. And, for susceptible people, there is mounting concern about a more than casual link between sugar addiction and alcoholism.

So, should you drink? I don't know. I *do* know that for many people, it can completely derail a weight loss program, but for others it can be worked into the plan. Only you can decide which group you belong in.

A personal story about alcohol

Years ago, I worked with a young mother who, ten years earlier, had been "Centerfold of the Year" for one of the most famous men's magazines in the world. I'll call her Tracey. Now, a decade later, she was still a strikingly beautiful woman, able to turn heads when she walked into any room, but . . . she was heavy. Her face was always just a tad bloated, she had a lot of creeping "spread" around her thighs and butt and stomach, and she was very self-conscious about the noticeable difference between how she looked in her heyday and her current condition. During the better part of a year we tried a lot of different approaches, different workout routines, different diets. She stayed relatively fit and kept from gaining any weight, but nothing we did really made much of a difference in her body. Ultimately, she moved away and I lost touch with her.

A year later, I was taping something in a television studio, and unexpectedly, much to my delight, there was Tracey. At first, I didn't recognize her. She looked like she had just stepped off the cover of a fitness video. She was tan and lean, sleek and muscled, and she looked content and glowing. I was absolutely dumbstruck by the change.

"Tracey," I said, "you look absolutely amazing. What kind of workout program are you doing?"

"Basically the same stuff I was doing before," she said.

"Well then," I asked, "what diet did you go on?"

"No diet really," she said, smiling. "I'm watching what I eat, but it's not a whole lot different than when you knew me."

"OK, I give up," I said, completely bemused. "What happened? What did you do?"

"Simple," she said. "I stopped drinking."

Food for thought.

• In conclusion, *eat from the As, limit (or eliminate) the Bs, and watch the Cs carefully.* To the extent that you do that, you will get the wonderful results that can be yours by following this plan. Not only will you lose unwanted fat, but you will probably find that you feel better than you have in years.

The Joy of Soy?

I'm more than a bit cautious about getting on the joy of soy bandwagon. I'm not a fan of the wholesale and uncritical use of all soy products, including powders, "health" bars and especially supplements. Like so much that is controversial in the nutrition community, the case of soy says a lot about marketing, economics and the American propensity for getting our information in sound bytes.

On the one hand, it does appear that the isoflavones (plant-based compounds found in soy) have unique properties, one of which is that they are anti-cancer. So far, so good. Some studies have shown a role for soy in the lowering of cholesterol and the prevention of coronary artery disease (which are *not* necessarily the same thing, may I point out). On the other hand, we have been very misled about both the *amount* of soy in the Asian diet and the *form* of soy in the Asian diet. Most Asian diets use soy as a condiment, in relatively small amounts and surrounded by sea vegetables, fish and green tea. And I think the syllogism "Asians have less heart disease, Asians eat more soy, therefore more soy equals less heart disease" is both simplistic and incorrect. (About 50 percent of all men in Japan also smoke cigarettes, but no one is selling us that as a health concept.) I'd be very surprised if it turned out that soy was the one element in the Asian diet that turned out to be the magic bullet, but I guess soy is a lot easier to market (and a lot more profitable) than fish and vegetables.

Here are a few points worth considering before you make soy products your one and only source of protein:

1. Soy contains goitrogenic compounds—compounds which undermine the healthy functioning of the thyroid gland. As Dr. Harold Kristal points out, "Sub-clinical hypothyroidism is already such a common health problem that caution is certainly warranted."
2. Soy products contain a number of "anti-nutrients." Chief among them are enzyme inhibitors that block the action of trypsin and other enzymes that you need to digest protein properly.
3. Soy is not a complete protein. It is missing methionine, which is an essential amino acid. If soy is your main source of protein, you will almost certainly not be getting enough B-12, which is hard enough for adults to absorb in any case, even from animal foods.
4. Soy contains phytic acid, which binds with calcium, zinc, iron and magnesium and reduces their bioavailability. Now interestingly, phytic acid is one of those compounds that can cut both ways—it binds to iron and to toxic metals, helping to decrease their concentrations, which is a good thing; on the other hand it does the same thing to zinc, which is not so good. Just something to consider.

The healthiest soy products are the fermented ones like tempeh and miso, which don't have any of the problems mentioned above, but they are not the ones we're eating the most of. In addition, for what it's worth, most of the soybeans currently being produced in the United States are genetically engineered, the implications of which have not yet been fully understood by anyone.

Probably most important, the phytoestrogens in soy—those compounds so touted for their health benefits—are actually a mixed blessing. Yes, they are weaker than "real" estrogen, and yes, they bind to the estrogen receptors in your body, which partially prevents the body's own estrogen from binding to those sites and possibly causing mischief. But—and this is a big but—the whole beauty of phytoestrogens is that they are weaker than "real" estrogen and, by occupying the "parking spots" for estrogen, can theoretically help reduce the downside of estrogen (breast cancer, for example). Doesn't it make sense to consider whether or not that benefit might be washed away by consuming so much of the phytoestrogens that you might as well be taking the real thing?

The problem with soy is not so much a problem with soy per se as it is a problem with the old American propensity for thinking "if *some* is good, a *hundred times that* is better." It's one thing to get a reasonable dose of isoflavones—such as genistein—from soy. It's quite another to take isolated supplements of these compounds in amounts several hundred times what is found in the food. In high amounts, isoflavones may have negative effects on other hormones (like thyroid) and taking hundreds of times the dosage of a weaker estrogen might well be erasing the benefits of phytoestrogens in the first place. And who really knows what the cumulative effect of having this much phytoestrogen exposure in our food supply has had on sexual maturity and development in young people?

I think for now the safest bet is to include soy products if you like, but not to depend on them exclusively. I still believe that it's a mistake to get all of your protein from soy and that a better choice would be to get your protein from a mix of soy and animal products such as eggs. I still like whey protein better for its completeness, its absorbability and its effect on the immune system (it increases the production of glutathione, one of the most important antioxidants in the body), but you could make a wonderful protein powder by mixing some soy protein powder in with your whey. Soy can absolutely be part of a healthy diet, especially soy from fermented products like tempeh and miso, and it can be used in a way that supports all kinds of good things, including weight loss. But for right now, I don't think we should eat unlimited amounts of it, and I definitely don't think we should be taking supplements of concentrated isoflavones.

A Word About Preparation Methods

Anything broiled or baked goes on the "A" list. Anything fried—anything at all, including but not limited to french fries, chicken, and fish—is serious "B" list material. This stuff is not only "fattening," it's health-destroying. No ifs, ands, buts, or political correctness. Sorry.

To maximize the health benefits of your Shape Up plan, I strongly suggest you include some raw foods on a daily basis. I'm talking here about fruits, nuts, seeds, and especially vegetables. Great examples: carrots, celery, peppers, onions, tomatoes, lettuces, spinach, apples, pears, plums, berries, raw cashews, and pumpkin seeds. Preferably as fresh as possible. Raw foods are loaded with enzymes and have what could unscientifically (but accurately) be called great "life force" in them. There are people who live on nothing but raw foods. While this may be too extreme, I do think you should try to eat some raw foods every single day. (One favorite of mine: tomatoes and bell peppers nicely seasoned with a dollop of extra virgin olive oil, lemon, and pepper.) Fresh vegetable juices count. Be creative.

How Often Should I Eat?

Regarding eating and the spacing of meals (or snacks), the basic concept is this: You want to keep your blood sugar even throughout the day so that you don't experience high peaks and low valleys of energy. You generally don't want to go too long without eating because your body goes into a kind of starvation mode—it thinks there's a famine, so it gets very good at creating storage fat, and the metabolism slows down as a survival tactic (kind of like turning down the thermostat when you're trying to conserve energy during a fuel shortage). In addition, on a practical level, when you go a real long time without eating, you generally feel famished and will eat anything that's put in front of you. Go seven hours without food before going out to dinner and most people will eat the basket that the bread comes in! For that reason alone it's not generally advisable to skip meals.

On the other hand, many people don't learn to respond to their body's internal cues and instead just eat because it's mealtime and there's food in front of them. One interesting study looked at the eating behavior of people who consistently flew back and forth from Europe to the United States and were always in different time zones (it's always mealtime *somewhere*). The study found that the travelers with weight problems ate whenever it was meal time, while the leanest travelers ate when they were hungry. In other words, the former group paid attention only to external and social cues, while the latter had learned to self-monitor a lot more effectively. In the ideal situation, you want to have small meals (or feedings) fairly frequently (every three to four hours) throughout the day. Small meals keep you from being too full and tired, from consuming more calories than you can use and from being on a blood sugar roller coaster.

So the real answer is to learn to listen to your body, eat when you are hungry and not go too long (more than four hours) without any food. And to eat the right stuff when you do eat. For most people this means eating at "mealtimes" plus a couple of nutritious snacks during the day, but for some people it can be accomplished with only three feedings. Mealtimes are merely conventions—learn the concepts of steady feeding, even blood sugar, sustained energy, listening to your body, and you can apply them any way you like.

SUPPLEMENTS

I'm often asked if I "believe" in vitamins, which, to me, is like asking, "Do you believe in air?" Vitamins and minerals are essential to life. You can choose to "believe" in them or not, but your body won't function properly without them.

What people usually mean when they ask that question is "Do you believe in *supplements*?" And the answer is, unequivocably, yes.

Here's why: Supplements are nothing more than a *delivery system* for nutrients, nutrients that were once abundant in our "factory-specified" diet but are increasingly hard to get in therapeutic and protective amounts from our current food supply. Can you live without them? Of course. You can also live without electricity and indoor plumbing. But now that it's available, why in heaven's name would you want to?

The American Dietetic Association and other conservative forces in the nutrition establishment would have you believe that you can get "all you need from food." Quite frankly, this is preposterous. The belief that you can get all you need from food is rooted in a very outdated view of the term "all you need." A little history will explain why.

In the early part of the twentieth century, a Polish chemist named Casimir Funk discovered that the anti-beriberi substance in polished rice was an amine (a nitrogen-containing compound). He proposed that this substance be named a "vital amine," a term which later became associated with a much larger class of nutrients (even though many of them were not amines at all). The term "vital amine" became shortened to "vitamin," and shortly afterwards, Funk and another researcher named Hopkins put forth the "vitamin deficiency theory of disease," which basically said that the absence of these vital substances caused diseases like scurvy (vitamin C), rickets (vitamin D), beriberi (thiamin) and pellegra (niacin). The RDA's and other "official" views of what we need in the way of vitamins and minerals continues to be referenced to this concept of "avoiding disease" rather than optimizing health.

I call this the "minimum wage theory" of nutrition. If by "all you need" you're talking about what's needed to prevent scurvy, rickets and the like, I'll concede that we don't need supplements. But I don't see much scurvy and beriberi around anymore. Overwhelming amounts of research have shown that vitamins and minerals in therapeutic dosages can reduce the risk for a multitude of diseases, protect the heart, strengthen the immune system, postpone the symptoms of Alzheimer's disease, decrease blood pressure, help with blood sugar control, reduce the incidence of certain birth defects like neural tube syndrome, improve brain function and memory, reduce the risk of cancer, improve symptoms of premenstrual syndrome, help modulate symptoms from allergies and asthma, help with intestinal dysbiosis and irritable bowel syndrome, protect the liver, and reduce stresses from environmental carcinogens. Can you get all you need for this level of optimal health and well-being from food alone?

Well, if you were living on a farm, rotating your crops, growing your own food organically, eating it fresh, hunting and eating wild animals that grazed on grass rather than grains and that you honored and respected as the American Indians did the animals they ate, and if you fished for game fish in fresh, uncontaminated waters, and if your level of stress was reduced by half, and if you were not exposed to smoke and environmental toxins, and if you didn't drink, use tobacco, eat sugar or refined foods or overuse antibiotics, well then maybe you could. But, as my father used to say, "If my grandmother had wheels, she'd be a wagon." The point is you *don't* do those things (if you do, please invite me to visit—I want to move to where you live!). Even in such an idyllic environment it might be hard to get enough vitamin E to have a therapeutic, protective effect on the heart, but on the other hand the heart wouldn't be under the same level of stress so perhaps you wouldn't need the same level of therapeutic protection.

The point is, take your supplements.

Recognizing that people differ widely in their inclination to take pills, even those that are good for them, I've created two different supplement programs. Level One is a basic entry-level supplement program that I would like to suggest that you consider taking as an absolute minimum. Level Two is a more comprehensive program that I believe will benefit just about everyone but requires that you pop a few more pills. In the best of all possible worlds, I'd like to see everyone in Shape Up on the Level Two program, but I'll settle for Level One for now! I think the health benefits are well worth the effort.

On a personal note, my wife Cassandra and I take well more than fifty of these a day, so we're used to it. We've made it into something of a morning ritual, so it's not only painless but actually part of something pleasant. It takes about five minutes to prepare some morning green tea with lemon and get the supplements ready for the day. Cassandra usually writes in her journal very early in the morning before going to work at the television studio, while I put our supplements together. We have a few moments together, celebrate the day, thank the universe for our lives and face the adventure that's sure to unfold. It takes only a few minutes, and has become something of a self-care routine that sets the tone for the rest of the day, and at the very least creates good energy with which to confront any little stumbling blocks that happen to come up. You can include it in a routine of your own making, but I promise you taking a few high-quality supplements to protect and ensure your health is not that big a deal and you can easily make it into a habit.

The Level One Shape Up Supplement Program

1. **A high-quality multimineral formula.** Minerals are easily as important as vitamins and are often overlooked. Although there has been an enormous amount of attention given to calcium, I'm actually much more concerned about magnesium. I believe the best research shows that at least 75 percent of women are deficient in this very important mineral, which is needed not only for bone health but for blood sugar control and a host of other important functions. If you are taking a "calcium-magnesium" formula, they should be in no less than a 2:1 ratio (at least half as much magnesium as calcium) and I wouldn't even mind a 1:1 ratio. Your multimineral should contain at least 400 mg of magnesium.

2. **A high-quality multivitamin formula.** Get the best you can find and afford. No matter what people tell you, there's a huge difference in quality from brand to brand. Why? Products vary with regard to the *freshness* of the ingredients, the *quality* of the ingredients (which form of the vitamins and minerals they use), the type and presence of fillers and binders, whether or not the product undergoes rigorous testing (assays) of representative batches for potency and quality (and how often) and how bioavailable and absorbable the final product is. I'm a big fan of the supplements made by the Designs for Health Institute, Metagenics, Cenegenics Medical Institute and the Life Extension Institute, but other brands are widely available and also very good (*see Appendix for contact information*). Supplement purchases should be taken seriously—don't just grab something off the supermarket, drugstore or even health food store shelf and assume it's good. There are huge differences among supplements—look for products from companies who know what they're doing and that are committed to quality.

It's going to be virtually impossible to get a good dosage of high-quality vitamins and/or minerals in one single pill. Most of the better brands will require that you take several to get the recommended dosage. There really isn't any way around this.

Your multivitamin should contain at least 50 mg of all of the B-complex vitamins, which, among other things, have been known to help many people feel more energetic as well as have better appetite control. Your multivitamin must contain at least 400mcg of folic acid, and I would prefer that you get 800 mcg.

3. **Fish oil capsules.** You're looking for a combination of two important fatty acids that we will discuss at length later on—EPA and DHA.

   As an alternative to fish oil capsules, you could buy a blended oil that contains the omega-3 fatty acids EPA and DHA in the right combination with an important omega-6 fatty acid called GLA (gamma-linolenic acid). GLA is found in evening primrose oil and borage oil, and women especially find this a helpful supplement especially prior to their periods. Three superb blended oils that I especially like are Essential Woman by Barlean's Organic Oils, Omega Plus by Omega Nutrition, and Udo's Choice by Flora, all widely available at health food stores. A couple of spoonfuls of any of these on a daily basis would be terrific. If you can stand it, cod liver oil is a perfectly good alternative (yes, Grandmother was right after all), but it doesn't contain any GLA.

4. **Chromium (400 mcg daily).** This trace mineral is next to impossible to get from a regular diet these days and is vitally important in managing blood sugar levels. Many studies have confirmed its value in a weight loss program, and even at much higher dosages, it has almost no downside. The chromium picolinate form is the most studied.

The Level Two Shape Up Supplement Program

1. A high-quality multimineral formula with at least 400 mg of magnesium.
2. A high-quality antioxidant formula.
3. B-complex.
   → Dividing your multiple into two formulas—an antioxidant formula and a B-complex—lets you concentrate on getting maximum antioxidant protection in the first, and a full spectrum

of high quality, good potency B vitamins in the second, rather than having to rely on getting both in the same formula, as is the case in Level One. The same caveats from Level One apply: Look for 50 mg of each of the Bs, and at least 400 mcg (preferably 800 mcg) of folic acid.

4. **Chromium.** (400 mcg daily)

5. **Fish Oil Capsules.**

6. **Vitamin C (500–3000 mg a day).** All the many, many documented reasons that you should supplement with this vitamin have been written about elsewhere—they're true.

7. **Vitamin E (400 IUs a day).** In the case of vitamin E, it really does make a difference that you get the natural form, which in this case means that on the label it will say, for example, "d-alpha-tocopherol," not the less effective synthetic "dl." Ask for a blend of mixed tocopherols.

8. **Digestive Enzymes:** For many reasons, most people can benefit from these, despite what the American Dietetic Association may think. Many clinicians feel that there is hardly a chronic ailment that doesn't have a digestive (or leaky gut) component, and many adults don't fully digest and absorb some proteins because of a lack of hydrochloric acid and digestive enzymes. Can't hurt, will probably help.

More on Supplements: A Second Line of Defense

For those who want to get even more into supplements, I recommend that you consider a few more "specialty" items.

Alpha lipoic acid. This is a nutrient that has the remarkable capacity to regenerate both vitamin E and vitamin C. It is a powerful antioxidant on which an enormous amount of research has been done, virtually all of it with positive results. Two conditions in which it is particularly indicated are diabetes (or blood sugar management in general) and liver health. The best book for the general public on alpha lipoic acid is *The Alpha Lipoic Acid Breakthrough,* by Burt Berkson, M.D., PhD. It is also covered in depth in *The Antioxidant Revolution,* by Lester Packer, Ph.D.

Saw palmetto oil. This remarkable herb has been found to be as effective as the prescription drug Proscar in treating benign prostate hyperplasia, which affects most men at some point in their lives. It helps prevent the conversion of testosterone to di-hydro-testosterone, and can help relieve the annoying symptoms of BPH. It's often found in "prostate" formulas with two other ingredients that are helpful for the prostate, nettles and pygeum. If you're a man over forty, I recommend taking it. If you're a woman and you love a man over forty, get it for him.

Folic acid. If you're doing either the Level One or the Level Two supplement program, you're getting the recommended amount of this nutrient, but it's worth mentioning why it's so important. For one thing, it has been shown definitively to prevent neural tube defects, so absolutely every woman who is of pregnancy age—whether she's planning to get pregnant or not—should be taking it. For another, it is one of those nutrients that are actually better absorbed when you get it from supplements than when you get it from food. Folic acid has also been used in formulas to treat depression and improve mood. Every nutritionist I respect thinks the recommended daily intake should be 800 mcg, but the government is keeping it at 400. Know why? Because if you have a B-12 deficiency (which is very serious stuff), folic acid intake can mask the symptoms. To me, the far more intelligent approach would be to make sure you take folic acid *and* B-12, but, hey, that's just me.

B-12. Yes, you're getting it in your multiple or in your B-complex, but B-12 can also be used therapeutically, away from the other B-vitamins, as a star in its own right. Long given by injection by nutritionally oriented M.D.'s, the oral form is not terribly well-absorbed by adults because of low levels of something in the stomach called "intrinsic factor," which is needed to make proper use of the B-12 you get from your food or supplements. Many people find that they have much more energy when they get proper amounts, and high-dose oral supplements (in the range of 1,000–2,500 mcg) seem to bypass the intrinsic factor problem somehow. The most absorbable form of B-12 is in meat, and with a reduction in meat consumption among many dieting and vegetarian women, plus an increase in antacid consumption (which causes a drop in stomach acid needed for absorption), very low intakes of B-12 are not uncommon. We used to believe that B-12 deficiencies (or sub-clinical deficiencies) were common only in older people, but a recent study at Tufts University showed that adults in their twenties, thirties, and forties were equally likely to be deficient. If you want to experiment with a therapeutic dose of B-12, take it at a different time from when you take your other vitamins. Many people notice a difference.

Milk thistle (or silymarin). The smooth operation of the detoxification pathways in the body are a vital part of good health, and that means that the liver—the major organ of detoxification—needs all the support it can get. This herb has been shown to protect liver cells and may help with detoxification in general. Detoxification is already one of the hottest topics in nutritional medicine and will continue to be as our bodies are now exposed to unprecedented amounts of toxins from both the environment and the food supply. Herbs like milk thistle—and dandelion root, another liver-friendly herb—can only help.

And if you don't eat red meat:

Take at least 1,000 mg of L-carnitine per day. This nutrient, often lacking in the diet, is necessary to get fat into the mitochondria of the cells, where it is burned for energy. Many experts believe that we don't get enough carnitine in the diet. Since red meat is the best source of it, those who don't eat meat should almost certainly take this supplement.

Should I ask my doctor about nutrition and supplements?

Asking your average doctor for information about nutrition is like asking your accountant for information about tennis. Your accountant might actually be a terrific tennis player—maybe he played in college and spends his weekends on the competitive club circuit—but if this is the case, it's a complete coincidence, and he certainly didn't learn how to play in accounting school.

Don't get me wrong. Some of my best professional friends are doctors. I talk to doctors every day. They are all-around invaluable sources of information. The doctors I speak with are some of the best-informed, most brilliant practitioners of nutritional medicine on the planet and have forgotten more about the clinical use of supplements than most people will ever know. They are particularly expert in knowing the interactions of pharmaceuticals, herbs, and supplements, and have a unique ability to combine science, intuition, clinical observation, and research in the time-honored tradition of empirical—rather than deductive—medicine.

And every one of them will tell you this: Everything they learned about nutrition they learned on their own. Every one. There is not an M.D. I know who claims to have learned anything of any use about the above-mentioned subjects in medical school. When it comes to food and nutrition, most of them basically learned what your average sixth grader learns in a home economics class. My doctor pals will also be the first to tell you that not only did they learn what they learned outside the general medical education model, but they encountered—and still encounter on a daily basis—virulent resistance to their integrative approach by the keepers of the cultish flame that is conventional medicine, aided and abetted by the pharmaceutical companies that have just a wee bit of a vested interest in keeping drugs and only drugs the treatment of choice for any condition on the planet.

It may be difficult to find an M.D. who knows and accepts the profound role that nutrients have on human health, and who knows how to use them therapeutically, but if you can find one, it will be worth the time spent looking.

What are the best supplements for weight loss?

I'm tempted to say "There aren't any," but that would be an oversimplification. I do think there aren't any that produce dramatic results. That said, I also think that if your nutritional status is less than optimal, all of your metabolic processes (including the "burning" of fat) are going to be compromised, so it's very important to make sure you're getting everything in optimal dosages, and that's where supplements can make a difference.

Chromium will help insulin do its job better, so it's on the top of my recommended list. Carnitine is often lacking in the diet and is important for fat burning; I wish we had more actual research on its effect on weight loss, but there is so much anecdotal and clinical experience indicating that it's helpful that it's hard not to include it in the recommended list. Many people seem to do better on higher dosages of the B vitamins.

I'm on the fence about such things as hydroxy-citrate, which some people claim help curb appetite; other claims for it include its reported ability to interfere with some of the conversion of carbohydrate to storage fat. I'm just not sure. Pyruvate has a lot of claims made for it, but only one good research study that I know of, and that one used an awful lot of pyruvate, more than most people would find palatable. CLA (conjugated linoleic acid) shows promise, but my experience with it is that sometimes it works, sometimes it doesn't. (It does, however, have other very real health benefits.)

In my opinion, nothing works as well as a moderate calorie, low-carbohydrate diet heavily weighted toward natural foods and fats, plenty of water, daily exercise and optimal general supplementation. I've yet to see a "fat burner" formula that really did very much.

"Fat Blocker" Drugs

When the announcement first came out that the FDA had approved Orlistat, a "fat-blocking, anti-obesity" drug marketed under the trade name Xenical, it was greeted with enthusiasm by the many sections of the public who, understandably, continue to hope that modern science will soon come up with a technology that will make losing fat easier and more painless than those oh-so-annoying "lifestyle changes." Read the sound bytes and do the auditory equivalent of squinting and you might easily draw the conclusion that Xenical lets you continue to point your car tires at the Golden Arches while painlessly melting away the tires around your waist. But if you read the reports a little more carefully, you might want to think twice before running out and searching for a doc who will prescribe it for you.

Xenical works in the gastro-intestinal tract by blocking the action of a fat-digesting enzyme. About one-third of the fat someone eats will, instead of being digested, accumulate in the intestines and be excreted.

Now that you know how it works, the first problem with using Xenical for fat reduction should be immediately apparent: It does nothing to the fat you've already accumulated. Since it works only on incoming fat in the diet, preventing only a percentage of it from going to your hips, it might, at best, slightly decrease the consequences of continuous bad eating.

But even this is not 100 percent clear, nor does it come without a price.

For one thing, by blocking the absorption of fat, the drug also interferes with the absorption of the all-important vitamins A, D, E, and K, as well as beta-carotene, all of which are fat-soluble. For another, Xenical is known for producing side effects like flatulence and bloating and, most famously, what is euphemistically referred to as "anal leakage."

The drug was approved only for "seriously overweight" people who meet the government's "more than 30 percent overweight" standard for obesity or for those who have diabetes, hypertension, or high cholesterol *and* are 20 percent overweight. That little detail won't stop people who don't fit the profile from demanding it, and we can be pretty sure that there'll be no shortage of doctors willing to prescribe it for them.

Even in clinical trials the results were pretty underwhelming: In one study, there was only a 4 percent difference in body weight between the group taking the placebo and the group taking the drug. And in another experiment reported in the *Journal of the American Medical Association*, many people who were taking Orlistat began to gain weight back after a year, even while continuing to take the drug.

Magic bullet? Sorry.

What's interesting to me is that the health food industry has long had a product out on the market that works in basically the same exact way. It's called "chitosan" and it too works by preventing the absorption of some of the fat in the diet. According to Earl Mindell, a leading authority on supplements, "[As chitosan] passes through the digestive tract it can absorb four to six times its weight in fat, thereby flushing it out of the body before it can be metabolized and stored as excess pounds." But because it has the same problems as Orlistat, I don't think it's a major player in the weightloss field, and the same caveats ("anal leakage," anyone?) apply.

Undoubtedly there are people who might benefit from drugs for weight loss, but there's little doubt in my mind that even if you are one of them, a Shape Up–friendly dietary program will only help things along.

What's the story with those metabolic enhancers?

The most common ingredient in "metabolic enhancers" is ephedra. Ephedra is basically legal speed. While I'd be lying if I said it's as dangerous as crack cocaine, a small dose is approximately equal to a few cups of strong coffee. Same deal with ma huang. These substances should be avoided like the black plague if you have any problems with high blood pressure. They can—and usually do—make you jittery, nervous and speedy, and they can raise blood pressure and heart rate. This does indeed temporarily speed up the metabolic rate, but how much that transfers to actual weight loss is anyone's guess.

These products will rev up the engine slightly—but without a lot of exercise to burn that gas, you're just producing a few extra calories as heat while doing some potential damage to the rest of your system. Except for the appetite effect (which would make you eat less—but so would diet pills)—the effect they have on calorie expenditure and fat loss pales when compared to exercise, muscle building and a diet designed to keep insulin levels from soaring into the stratosphere.

Other ingredients often found in some of these products, besides the stimulants, are carnitine and chromium, which I discuss in this chapter. I believe both of them play an important part in supporting different aspects of metabolic function (blood sugar in the case of chromium, and fat metabolism in the case of carnitine). But the amounts in the metabolic enhancers is usually far less than what's needed, and if you want them you can do better getting them as separate products from reputable companies.

Want my opinion? When it comes to metabolic enhancers, step away from the kiosk, throw out the sugar and the high-carb junk and head toward the gym.

EXERCISE

Exercise and the Shape Up Program

The Shape Up exercise program consists of two simple components: *walking* and *strength training*. In week one, you'll begin the walking program. In week two, you'll be adding the first of the strength training exercises. From then on, we'll be adding exercises to our workout routine on a week by week basis. (*Remember, the exercise component of the Shape Up program is designed for beginners; if you're already an intermediate or advanced exerciser, go to the Appendix for your weekly program.*)

It will help to have a pair of light dumbbells, but if you don't have them, you can do the dumbbell exercises with a couple of bottles of water, or you can eliminate the added weight altogether.

Sets and Reps: How Much Should I Do?

If you're new to this terminology, here are some quick definitions. (They're not nearly as complicated as you might think.) Any exercise movement has a start point and a finish point that are usually the same. For example, if you stand outside your front door, and then walk around the block till you get back to your front door, you will have started and finished in the same spot, and you will have performed one repetition (or "rep") of the exercise called "walking around your block." Repetitions are grouped into "sets." A set can contain anywhere from two or three repetitions to (in some advanced specialty exercise programs) as many as 100. (Don't worry, we won't be doing any sets of 100 reps.)

Since the premise of this whole program is that you start where you are right now, the number of reps and sets you do is going to be determined by your current fitness level. I'm going to give you guidelines, but don't let them scare you off. For example, with some of these exercises, you may find that you can only perform one repetition. That's fine. That's *your* personal starting point. The next time you do it, you'll add another. The sets and reps are just guidelines, goals to work up to. Some of you may find them to be too easy. That's great too. Add another set, or if it's a weight-bearing exercise, add a few more pounds. Remember that this is *your* program, and the only "perfect" way to do it is the way that works best for you.

Finding Time for Exercise

> The choice may have been mistaken. . .
> the choosing was not.
>
> — *STEPHEN SONDHEIM*
> (*FROM* SUNDAY IN THE PARK WITH GEORGE)

If I had to make my list of the top-ten problems people have with starting a program, finding time for exercise would definitely be at the top of it. But here's the thing: If you're looking to find some spare time when you can fit exercise in, forget about it. We're living in the early part of the twenty-first century. *No one* has spare time. It's like "spare money." You can choose to budget money and time any way you want, but none of it is extra, none of it is spare.

Time is the great equalizer. The poorest person on the planet and the richest have exactly the same amount of it: twenty-four hours per day. No more, no less. So let's forget about finding extra time. (Where are you gonna find it, under a rock?) Instead, let's talk about developing a budget. Let's talk about creating our life the way we want it to be.

As a writer, I'm always fascinated with what the writing process is like for other writers. Writing is right up there with exercise in the procrastination sweepstakes. There are thousands of failed writers all over the place who are sure that the only reason they're not successful is that they "couldn't find time," or didn't have the right computer, or the right quiet room, or because they had too many other responsibilities. But successful writers—like successful exercisers—don't have any more minutes in the day than unsuccessful writers. My favorite writing story is the one about the lawyer who wrote a novel in the wee hours of the morning before proceeding to go to work, where he put in a sixty-hour week while supporting a family with three small children. It took him three years to complete the novel. The novel was *A Time to Kill*, and the lawyer was John Grisham.

Oh, and did I mention the almost destitute young housewife with a young child and a burning desire to write no matter what? She'd sit in coffee shops and write by longhand while the baby would nap. Did it for a long time, by the way, with very little support from the universe. Her name is J. K. Rowling. Maybe you know her. She wrote the Harry Potter books.

So let's dispel this notion of "I can't find the time." Of course you can't. Neither can I. The problem is not one of time, it's one of *habit development*. It's about taking something that you're not *used* to doing—exercise—and turning it into something that you're not used to doing *without*. Work on the plan for habit acquisition, and believe me, time will take care of itself.

So how do you build a habit?

Suppose you're playing catch with a little kid. A real little kid, one who can barely get her hands around the ball and is just learning to throw. What do you do? Do you throw the ball as hard and as fast as you can? Of course you don't, because it would be impossible for her to catch it, and she would get completely frustrated and give up. Watch a father teaching his kid to hit a baseball sometime. How does he pitch those first balls? Easy and gently. Underhand.

Now why do you do it like that?

Cause you want the kid to develop her skill. Because the one thing you don't want is for her to feel defeated. Because you don't want her to be frustrated. Because skill building has to start slowly, a little at a time. When she gets good at catching the ball with an easy throw, when he gets good at hitting the ball with an easy pitch, then you make it marginally harder. You keep the challenge level just slightly above the skill level, so that the skill can grow organically, step by step, and the learner is always reinforced positively with a feeling of accomplishment.

And why, at the risk of repeating the obvious, do we do it this way?

Well, if I can be blunt, because no one likes to do what they suck at. If you keep having an unsuccessful experience with something, you just stop doing it. It's not fun to fail. And that's what most people have done with their exercise programs. They cut off a big chunk right at the beginning, they can't chew it, and they spit it out. And they stop.

And blame it on not having enough time.

You are going to teach yourself something new, a new skill, a new habit, just as surely as you would teach a child to catch and throw a ball. If you start with some ridiculous goal like "I must do one hour of jogging every day," it will be like throwing a fastball to the kid who never played catch before. You're going to be frustrated, you're going to think you stink at this game, and you're going to give up. That you can take to the bank.

So you have to do something different. You have got to stack the deck in your own favor.

You have to set the game up so you win.

See, the subconscious mind is very simplistic. It's very digital. It knows two states: on or off. Win or lose. Success or failure. If you set yourself an initial goal like "thirty minutes on the treadmill" and you only do twenty-six minutes, whether you are aware of it or not, your subconscious mind logs that as a failure. You aimed for thirty and didn't make it. Somewhere in your subconscious is a little voice sticking out its symbolic tongue and yelling "*loser!*" But if you set a goal of *five* minutes, and you *do* five minutes, guess what? Your mind logs that as a *win*. Which it is. Does it matter that it's "only" five minutes? Not on your life. What matters is that you had a positive experience.

In the first months of exercise, all we're trying to do is to log those positives. We're in habit-building mode, not in "how much exercise did I do?" mode. It is not important how *much* you do—what is important is that you do *something*. Consistently. That's how we build a habit successfully. That's why the intro level Shape Up program begins with only ten minutes of walking three times a week. What you're really trying to do here is condition your subconscious. You want to trick it into thinking that exercise is always a "win" situation for you. Maybe for you, right now, that means just doing five minutes a day. No problem. Your conscious mind may be saying, "But five minutes can't possibly make any difference," but it's dead wrong. What makes a difference—and believe me, this is the most important difference of all—is that you keep your word to yourself. You *said* you would do five minutes . . . and you *did* five minutes. You *said* you're going to walk half a block . . . and you *walked* half a block. It may not seem like much, but on a subconscious level you were learning the most valuable lesson in habit development: You're learning to believe your own word.

You're learning to believe that when you *say* something, it *happens*.

And that is truly the secret weapon of the entire Shape Up program.

I once trained a woman named Marnie, an absolutely lovely and charming occupational therapist who weighed around 250 pounds. She had never exercised successfully, hated the concept, didn't see how she could possibly fit it into her extraordinarily busy life, but had reluctantly come to the gym on doctor's orders. She had tried working out several times in the past and had been given long routines of weights and aerobics that she found both difficult and dull and had abandoned within a matter of days. She had very little hope that this would be different but had promised her doctor that she would give it one more shot.

The first training session, we did nothing but talk. I didn't even let her change into her gym clothes.

At the end of our meeting, I gave her her first assignment: Show up for the next session.

Which she did. Early, actually.

The second time we talked some more. What was her job like? Where did she want to be in a few years? What was her health like? How, if at all, did she feel her weight held her back? How did she feel about her body? You know, stuff like that.

The third time I showed her how the treadmill worked. She actually got on it, and we walked together on adjoining treadmills.

For three minutes.

Yes, you heard me right. Three minutes. And that was her assignment for the next two visits. *Three minutes on the treadmill.* No more, no less.

She had now logged in five successful trips to the gym. I upped her assignment to four minutes.

See where I'm going with this?

The biggest mistake people make when it comes to incorporating exercise into their lives is concentrating on the amount they do and how quickly it will produce results. It's the wrong focus. Until it becomes something you can't imagine living without, the focus should be simply on doing *something* consistently. Do you realize that if you started with as little as one minute a day and over the next two months added no more than thirty seconds each day, you'd be up to a half hour of daily exercise in sixty days? You can always up the ante once you develop the habit. The trick is developing the habit.

In case you're wondering what happened with Marnie, she became one of the strongest athletes I ever trained. When she finally left me to move out west, she was regularly lifting weights, running in Central Park, going mountain biking on weekends and looking forward to learning how to ski.

You can do it, too. Or any version of that that suits your life.

If exercise is new to you, treat this part of the program as a remedial course in the power of your word. Trust me that it does not matter how little you do right now. What matters is that you promise to do it, and then you keep that promise. Keep the bar low for now—in fact, I insist on it. You can always raise it. You *will* raise it.

When *you* say so.

But first you have to learn to negotiate this skill at the beginner's level, just like the little child learning to throw a ball. You have to believe in your own word again.

And if that little voice in your head tells you that a few minutes a day can't possibly make any difference, well then, please tell her she's more than welcome to her opinion, but to please stop chattering for a few minutes while you go work out.

A Personal Story

Argue for your limitations and they will be yours.

— RICHARD BACH

Whenever people tell me they have no time for exercise, I think of my dog Max.

For years, I thought it would be nice to have a dog. I'd see people walking in Central Park with their dogs, I'd run into people on the street with a new puppy, I'd visit friends who seemed to have great relationships with their pets, and it always seemed like such a cool thing, you know, you have this dog, and it provides companionship and unconditional love and it's a conversation starter on the street, and it looks really cool on a Christmas card picture.

But when I started to think about the responsibilities, I'd hear my mother's voice in my head saying the things she'd always said when I was a kid and begged for a puppy: Who's going to walk it? Who's going to take care of it? Who's going to feed it? Who's going to take it to the vet? It's cruel to have a dog in the city. . . . Well, you get the idea, it's not exactly a unique scenario.

I was working as a personal trainer. I was getting up at around 5:30 A.M., working back-to-back clients till around 10, running back to my apartment to write, going to the gym to work out, then back for more clients or a lecture preparation. I was living alone; a dog seemed like a really bad choice. It just couldn't be fitted in to my lifestyle.

Then one day, I really wanted a dog.

I mean *really*. Not just intellectually, not just as a concept. Maybe I was ready to take the intermediary step between solitary bachelorhood and reponsible connectedness. Who knows? I just remember that something shifted from the abstract "it would be nice if . . ." to a definite "this is something that needs to happen."

So I got Max, a sixteen-week-old Golden Retriever.

And I committed, without any evidence or support from the universe, mind you, that it was somehow going to work.

I had to get up a little earlier.

I found that there were some breaks in my day that I hadn't noticed before, when I could come home and walk him.

Neighbors who thought he was adorable started volunteering to babysit him.

I found a "doggie day care" center that I had never known existed right next to my gym, where I could leave Max for several hours at a time while he frolicked merrily with a new group of friends.

I discovered that a neighbor had a hidden courtyard and a dog of her own named Dice, who fell in love with Max. The neighbor presented us with a standing invitation for Max to come over and play while I was away training clients. She even gave me a key to the courtyard.

It's been nine years. Max has since been joined in my little family by Tigerlily, a Staffordshire bull terrier, Woodstock, a pit bull mix of undetermined origins, and Cassandra, a human.

What I learned from this is that even when circumstances seem to say "there is no way," the power of the human spirit can create one.

Getting Max was impractical. I could have gotten a ton of agreement that it was a bad idea. But once I knew I really needed to have a dog in my life, once I made that commitment to action, even in the absence of any promise of the universe to cooperate, doors began to open. Stuff began to show up. Opportunities presented themselves.

I get letters from people telling me how impossible their schedules are, how impossible it is for them to exercise. Sometimes a rundown of their daily activities and responsibilities gets me tired just reading it. It absolutely seems like there is no time in the day for anything else.

And if you believe that, if you believe there is *no way*, then guess what . . .

You'll be right.

But if sometimes, even in the absence of any evidence, even when circumstances seem impossible, you nonetheless commit . . . even before you've figured out how to do whatever it is you commit to . . .

. . . well then sometimes . . .

miracles happen.

THE TOOLS OF THE SHAPE UP PROGRAM

The Big Picture

Each week, you're going to be given assignments in each of five categories:

1. Journal
2. To-do list"
3. Food
4. Exercise
5. Self-assessment

These assignments will be short and easy, but you need to do all of them. They work together and the end result adds up to a lot more than the sum of the single parts.

I'm also going to ask you to write a contract with yourself, which I'll explain in a bit.

This program was developed on the Internet, where it was enormously successful in part because each week built upon the week before, and because there was so much support among the participants in the live chats and on the bulletin boards. In doing this program over the years, I've found that people can easily duplicate the experience at home on their own. It's not necessary that you have a buddy to do the program with, but if you can find one it would definitely help. It can be someone you see every day or it can be someone on-line that you've never met in person. Doesn't matter. The ability to have another "committed listener" who will be present for you and allow you to speak your commitments and intentions helps to make those commitments real in the universe and helps you—and the other person—practice keeping your word.

Each week on the Internet, we had a different topic for lecture and discussion. In this book the chapters that are interspersed between the weekly assignments are expanded versions of the material covered in those discussions. You can read each chapter as you come to it week by week, or you can read through the entire book now and go back to the assignments as needed.

The tools of this book are truly meant to be used, in some fashion, for the rest of your life. Keeping a journal, continuing to ask yourself some form of the self-evaluation questions, examining your life, eating consciously and building exercise sequentially are tools that will lead to self-knowledge and inner strength and will virtually guarantee you a powerful existence whatever path you choose. Diet books and exercise fads will undoubtedly come and go. The tools of this program will give you the ability to examine what works for you and the strength to trust what you find.

That will never go out of style.

The Journal: Much More Than a Food Diary

One of the most important tools in this program is the journal. You may be familiar with the concept if you've done food diaries before, but what I want you to do with this is a little bit different.

A lot different, actually.

You're going to record everything that you eat, just like in a regular food diary. Everything. Every morsel, every sip. If you have to ask "Does this count?" it does. And yes, you're probably going to hate this part. I feel this way every time I have to clean out a closet or an attic in which I've been stuffing boxes, pictures, old clothes, LPs from high school, trophies from camp, a non-functional Walkman I keep thinking I'll fix someday, magazines I thought I'd read, outdated textbooks from college and anything else I couldn't bring myself to throw out. But you know what? You can't clean that closet till you empty it. And unless you're willing to take all that stuff out and shine a bright, unforgiving (and nonjudgmental) light on the room, you'll never get it really clean. You'll just be straightening up the mess, doing damage control and hoping you can close the door for another year without the boxes of junk tumbling out.

So yes, you'll hate doing this. And, yes, you'll do it anyway. Why? Because you said so. And for no other reason. Not because I told you to, but because you said you would. (A big part of this program is about your finding out that you can keep your own word.) And here's the good part: You don't get to stop with simply writing down food portions. I want you to record your moods, your reactions, your feelings. And I promise you, you'll be having lots of those. You may be mad at me, you may think I'm a jerk for "making" you do this, you may be furious, sad, elated, melancholy, depressed, hopeless or ecstatic. Doesn't matter. Write it down. It doesn't have to be elaborate, just honest and spontaneous. Shorthand is fine. No points subtracted for penmanship or spelling. No one will ever see this but you, so if you want to rant and rave, go ahead. If you want to write a poem, I won't tell. Carry the journal with you everywhere. I want you to begin to discover the relationship between food and mood, so often concealed in our hectic lives. If you're feeling an unstoppable craving, I want to be able to link it up with what you ate, did or felt earlier. This whole program is about connecting the dots and making connections where before confusion reigned.

When you keep a food diary (or, more effectively, a journal), you're basically undertaking a project the sole purpose of which is to better understand *you*. The ancients believed that naming something allowed you to master it, or at least to understand it better. Journaling, in a way, lets you master the universe by using the power of your own voice, albeit through the written word. In our case, the universe we're attempting to master is that of our own bodies, but the possibility exists that we wind up mastering so much more.

Disc jockeys have a saying: *Play it and say it.* We journal keepers should adopt that saying but with a twist: *Say* it, and you'll *play* it. By constantly telling the truth, in the safe and private context of your own writing, you make your word law in the universe. Name it and you own it.

The journal helps you to crystallize what you're feeling and focus in on what is actually going on. Feelings are often diffuse, elusive, and hard to pinpoint. Separating "what happened" from the story we make up about it is easier when we write it down. (Think Sargeant Joe Friday in *Dragnet*: "Just the facts, ma'am, just the facts.") Always remember my favorite mantra: The facts don't make us miserable, the *meaning we attach to them* (our "stories") do. Once you truly understand the difference, you're well on the way to disempowering the self-destructive story and simply dealing with the truth rather the excess baggage you attach to it.

Food journals also have the more mundane purpose of letting us really see what goes into our mouth. Unconsciousness is the biggest enemy of success in weight loss. Most overeating—in fact, most *eating*—is unconscious. It's a mindless, habitual, conditioned reaction to a wide variety of cues, few of which have to do with hunger. By forcing them into consciousness by writing down what you're doing, when you're doing it, and how you're feeling at the time, you get the unprecedented opportunity to really examine what's what and to transform automatic behavior into that which comes from conscious choice.

Journals also let us begin to make connections between food and mood. One of the problems with the American diet is that we eat so much,of so many things, and our physical and emotional reactions to these foods are often so delayed, that we rarely get an opportunity to actually do the detective work that would lead us to discover the effects food have on our moods, energy levels and mental outlook. Similarly, by making room in the journal for notes about what was happening and what we were feeling, we can also bring into clear focus just what conditions are dangerous triggers for non-nurturing eating behaviors.

Finally, for many, the journal is one of the only places where we can really be alone with ourselves. Freed from the knowledge that someone else will see and judge what we're feeling and saying, many of us discover that it is truly possible to explore feelings, behaviors, fantasies and even "unacceptable" thoughts that we spend a great deal of psychic energy keeping hidden, not only from our loved ones but from ourselves. Freed from the constraints of social acceptability and "proper behavior," you're able to really delve into the deepest parts of yourself. The journal is your own private letter to yourself.

In ten years of practice, I've yet to meet someone who gave journaling an honest try and didn't get some benefit out of it, often a benefit that was wholly unexpected yet profoundly. The beautiful part of it is that there's no right way to do it. You can scrawl angry words on a page, "say" things to parents, husbands, loved ones that you've never been able to say, or just make a simple old list of what you're eating and when.

Remember, you can't throw out what's in that closet of yours till you're willing to take it out and look at it and see if it still fits your life. Throwing out stuff can be hard and is rarely an emotionally neutral act.

But if you do it, you create something that wasn't there before: space.

And in that space there's room for you to create something new.

And *that's* what the Shape Up program is about.

The To-do List: Dealing With Completion

Earlier, in Chapter 4, I asked you to make a short list of actions or tasks that you've been putting off that would make a difference to you if you completed them. Let's talk a little more about that list right now and how it's intimately connected with the success of this whole enterprise.

Many people don't discover how much psychic energy is drained from them by having dozens of "incompletes" hanging around in their lives until they actually start to clean some of them up. These incompletes are like open files on your computer that you're not using. They take up more and more space, eventually cluttering up the background so much that the computer begins to operate more sluggishly; eventually you get one of those awful "Not enough memory to complete task—close some programs and retry" messages.

If you made that list I asked you to make, you were probably able to come up with a barrelful of things that live so consistently on your permanent to-do list that they might as well be paying rent. Many of these are small and innocuous—annoying little tasks and errands, like making a phone call you've been putting off, paying the electric bill, returning a dress that didn't fit right, taking a movie back to the video store. Some, however, are a lot bigger—stuff that you've always wanted to do but never did (like finishing a college degree or writing a novel), stuff that you've been dreading (breaking off a destructive relationship, quitting a job, firing an employee), stuff that has never been resolved (cleaning up"some long-buried feelings about a parent or sibling, forgiving a transgression). In other words, stuff that lives on the side streets of your mind but takes up space nonetheless, even though you may only be conscious of it at odd times when someone or something pushes the mental button that dusts off the file and brings it out of the stacks and into the light.

Now what do all these things have to do with losing weight?

Well, as it turns out, a lot.

To prove it, let me give you an example.

Let's say you had a friend who told you she was going to meet you for lunch at 1 P.M., and she showed up at 1:30, breathless, apologetic, explaining that the traffic was just *impossible*. You'd probably be irritated but get over it. Suppose, now, that you make a second date with her a week later, and *again* she shows up thirty minutes late, this time telling you that she forgot her keys and had to go back to her office to pick them up before coming to meet you. And she's *so* sorry. The *next* time, the taxi had a flat tire. Time after *that* the subway got delayed.

Each time she tells you that it absolutely won't happen again, that no matter *what* she's going to be on time, that she won't let anything stand in the way of keeping this appointment, and to *please* give her one more chance.

So you make one more lunch date.

And she shows up half an hour late.

OK, think. What's happened to your friend's credibility? Will you ever believe in her ability or willingness to be on time? Or has she lost all credibility with you—has she become someone whose word means nothing, and who can't be believed or counted on (at least not when it comes to punctuality and lunch dates)?

Well, when it comes to dieting and weight loss, most of us are exactly like that friend. We have promised ourselves that we'll start tomorrow so many times, we've gone on so many dietary wild goose chases, we've made so many forgotten New Year's resolutions and broken so many solemn vows that we have lost credibility *in our own eyes*. We have stopped taking what we say to ourselves seriously.

We no longer believe our own word.

When that happens, a very important link between *intention* and *behavior* is broken, and with that break comes the loss of a sense of our own power to make things happen. Our word is no longer meaningful. We no longer believe we have the ability to follow through and make stuff happen.

Although this plays out in weight loss in a big and obvious way, it also shows up in a lot of small, insignificant places as well. Like the phone call we keep promising to make. The closet we keep meaning to clean out. The book we keep saying we're going to read. The class we keep meaning to sign up for.

The weight we keep promising to lose.

So this to-do list is really about *completion*. It's about relearning your power in the universe. Things become so *because you say so*. You get to experience the connection between your *saying* something is going to happen and it actually *happening*. It's a heady feeling, and there's nothing more empowering.

With this in mind, I want you to revisit that task list you began in Chapter 4. No task or errand is too small to include. What's important here is not the of the task, but the fact that you *say* you're going to do it, and then you get it done. That you begin healing and rebuilding the lost power of your own word.

When you find yourself adding really big stuff to that list of incomplete tasks or actions, I want you to break it down into smaller steps, concrete, specific actions that you can take action on and then check off the list, one at a time. For example, let's say that you've been promising yourself you're going to go back to school and get a nursing degree but you've never gotten around to it. Sketch out an action plan, step by step, that relates to that specific goal. The first step might be to make one phone call to the college to get a catalogue and application. The second step might be to fill it out. The third might be to have a conversation with someone who can advise you about financial aid. (This, by the way, is great practice for the skill of losing weight *one pound at a time*. The absence of this skill defeats many people who see their weight loss as such a huge project that they give up before even starting.) The idea here is to have specific, manageable action goals that you can complete and check off, making this a *game at which you can actually win*. Remember, the goal here is to rehabilitate the connection between your word and reality. Like all rehabilitations, it takes time, but you can cover an amazing distance if you're willing to tackle it one small step at a time.

You can continue to add to (and subtract from, as you check them off) this master task list throughout the program.

The Self-Assessment Questions

As part of each week's assignment, there will be a series of questions I want you to answer. At first you may not see the relevance of these questions to weight loss or the point of doing them. Here's where I'm going to ask for your trust. You don't need to understand, right now, why answering these questions is part of the weekly assignment. Just do it.

What you do need to understand, though, is that no one has ever lost weight—not in our society, anyway—without it having some meaning or impact on the rest of their life. Whether it's ten pounds or more than a hundred, it's just not possible for most people to transform their bodies unconsciously. And anything that takes effort has meaning in our lives. We feel victory when we do it and defeat when we don't. We make all kinds of decisions about what we're made of based on whether we can or can't do it. We let it determine if we feel attractive, accomplished, sexy, important, successful, glamorous. People have very strong feelings about their weight and their bodies and what that weight means.

In that context, I'm going to ask you some questions each week about what's going on with you. Some of them have to do with weight, some may seem like they don't. Answer them anyway. You won't fully understand the point of the exercise till you do it—and that's because the point is different for each person. People get very different things out of doing this work, but rarely do they think, at the end of the day, that it's been a waste of time.

So every week as part of your assignment, I'm going to ask you to answer a couple of questions in your journal. These questions are an opportunity for you to think, feel and reflect on where you are in your life at a given moment in time. Spend some time with them. Let your "right brain" play around. See what comes up. There's no right way to do this exercise. The questions were designed to facilitate a process which can help you get clearer about bpth the things you really want, and the things that are in the way of getting what you want. Think of it as a way to shine a flashlight into some corners of those closets we talked about cleaning out—maybe you'll rediscover some gems there that you'd forgotten all about, or maybe you'll see how some stale old ideas might be taking up unnecessary space and holding you back from going where you want to go. Consider this part of the homework—like your life (and your weight)—a work in progress. It might be interesting to write your answers in now, however they come to you, and then answer some of the same questions again at the end of the program, or even a few months (or years) from now.

It's interesting to watch how this exercise unfolds in time. Sometimes what looks like success to you at one point in time has a way of growing as you expand your horizons and start believing in yourself more. As an example, read the following passage from an autobiographical work in which the author discusses his dreams and hopes for a successful life. See if you can guess who wrote it before looking at the answer.

Oh, I had big dreams back then.

I would live in a one-bedroom condo just off the Strip, complete with cable and a leather couch that I would pick out myself. I'd even put some money down and get one of those great new Sony Beta machines that had just come out. I'd be able to buy new clothes from the mall instead of having to wear only the clothes I got for Christmas and my birthday all the time. And when I went to the casinos, I'd drive my brand-new used Datsun Z into the valet, tipping the kid a five-dollar bill without even blinking. If I wanted a sandwich at the coffee shop, I'd just buy it. I'd buy beer by the bottle instead of draft . . . I was going to be big, big, big!

Think for a minute about the person who might have written that. I'll give you a hint. At the time, he was a bartender in Las Vegas, hoping against hope to become a moderately successful comic on the comedy club circuit.

Give up?

His name is Drew Carey.

The point is, whatever your goals and dreams are right now, write them down, but be willing to be surprised at how life unfolds. Those dreams and goals of yours are fluid, not static, and more than you know they are a product of what you *believe you can achieve* and what you *believe you deserve*. You may be surprised at how differently you feel about things one year down the road.

The first step, however, is being specific about what you want to achieve *right now*. That goes for changing your body as well as your life. Just be specific about what you want, and adhere to the old adage: Keep your eyes on the stars and your feet on the ground.

Staying in the Game: The Contract

One of the most frequently asked questions of anyone undertaking a body renovation program like the Shape-Up is this: How do I stay motivated?

I'm always amused by the answers most diet gurus give to this question. It's usually some amalgam of self-help, motivational tips, cheerleading and positive thinking that often reminds me of a football coach at halftime. Why do I say I'm amused by it?

Well, because I have a very different take on the issue of motivation.

See, motivation really just means desire. You don't have any shortage of motivation. You have plenty of *desire* to shape up; you would *love* to have a new and improved body and a higher level of health and energy and vitality. The problem is *remembering* that when it's competing with a *different* set of desires. When we're stressed, tired, frustrated, angry, confused or despairing, the desire to lose weight and get in shape seems to fade into the background, and a *new* desire comes to the foreground. At that point in time the main thing you're motivated to do is *feel better now*. When chocolates beckon at the end of a stress-filled day, and the rewards of the Shape Up program seem remote, the contest between the two sets of motivations is a mismatch. You need some help. You need someone to speak for the part of you that wanted to make some changes in the first place.

So let's reframe the question. We probably don't need to be asking, "How can I stay motivated to lose weight?" because that is just another way of asking "How can I keep *wanting* to lose weight?" A better question would be this: How can I even the odds so that my *motivation to lose weight* (and feel better in the long run) has a fighting chance against my *motivation to feel better in the moment*?

So basically, all questions about staying motivated really come down to this: You've got two coaches shouting in your ear, one saying "*Go for the gold*" and one saying "*Feel better now: sit down and relax!*" Which one are you going to listen to?

Stella Adler, the great acting teacher, used to tell her pupils the following: "You all have little voices, little trolls sitting on your shoulder, chattering away in your ear. These voices tell you that you're a terrible actor, that you have no business going on stage, that you're going to be found out any minute and you will be exposed as the failure you are. *If you wait for that chatter in your ear to stop, you will never act.* What you must do is look over to the troll, and say, 'now listen here, mister. You can stay there, but you'll have to stop chattering for a moment while I go on stage and act!'"

Every one of us has these little voices in our heads, which I like to imagine looking like the famous cartoon that shows a man with a devil whispering into his left ear and an angel whispering into his right ear. (The only difference among people, I believe, is in how loudly the voices speak and on what subjects.) You will never silence their chatter completely. The real action is in learning how to live with them and not to give them so much power.

Learning to disempower the negative voices is an important part of mastering both life and weight loss. And here's where it gets tricky. See, at times when you most need her, your "angel" voice doesn't get the microphone. The motivation to lose weight and feel better in the long run doesn't speak as loudly as the motivation to feel comforted *right now*. At those end-of-the-day periods when you're craving stuff that's going to take you off your Shape Up plan, or when you're stressed out from a fight with your boyfriend/lover/husband/wife, or depressed about a bad day at work, or burned out, or bored, or any of the myriad of other situations that make eating the wrong stuff easy, the voice of the "devil troll" gets turned up full volume. Here are some of the things she says:

"Oh, you deserve it after that day you've had!"

"It's not going to make any difference anyway!"

"One won't kill you."

"You'll always be fat, so why bother?"

"You can start tomorrow."

Sound familiar?

It gets worse.

At these times, the angel troll gets laryngitis. Whatever you said you were going to do, whatever you gave your word on, somehow gets lost in all the shouting. The "devil troll" has the microphone, and the crowd is cheering her on. As Susan Estrich, the attorney who wrote the excellent book *Making the Case for Yourself*, says, you have, at that moment, no one to speak for you.

Hence, this tool.

To give yourself every advantage during those tricky make or break times, you're going to prepare a *contract*. The contract is between you and you. The only thing you have to do—one of the few things you have to do in this program to make it work—is to make the following promise: Reread the contract before breaking your word.

Oh, and one more thing. Neither of those two warring "voices," those two sets of motivation, is *inherently* stronger or weaker than the other. Not only that, neither of them is *inherently* good or bad. The only thing that makes one of them "win" is this: *You chose it.* You gave your word, and your word is *the only thing* that gives one of the voices more power than the other.

And to help you remember that, here's the contract.

Write it out in longhand and put it in your journal.

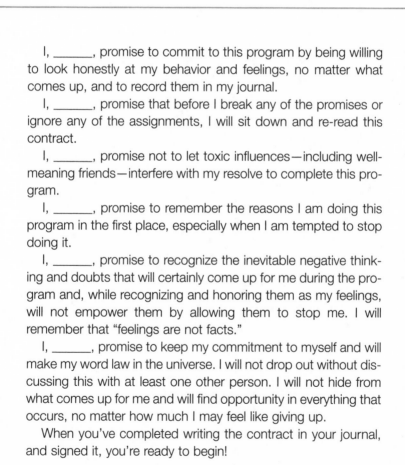

I, _____, promise to commit to this program by being willing to look honestly at my behavior and feelings, no matter what comes up, and to record them in my journal.

I, _____, promise that before I break any of the promises or ignore any of the assignments, I will sit down and re-read this contract.

I, _____, promise not to let toxic influences—including well-meaning friends—interfere with my resolve to complete this program.

I, _____, promise to remember the reasons I am doing this program in the first place, especially when I am tempted to stop doing it.

I, _____, promise to recognize the inevitable negative thinking and doubts that will certainly come up for me during the program and, while recognizing and honoring them as my feelings, will not empower them by allowing them to stop me. I will remember that "feelings are not facts."

I, _____, promise to keep my commitment to myself and will make my word law in the universe. I will not drop out without discussing this with at least one other person. I will not hide from what comes up for me and will find opportunity in everything that occurs, no matter how much I may feel like giving up.

When you've completed writing the contract in your journal, and signed it, you're ready to begin!

WEEKS ONE AND TWO

Week One

Week One: Journal

If you haven't already done so, get your journal and begin writing in it. At the very least, begin keeping a record of the food you eat. Remember, this includes *everything*.

Week One: To-Do List

- Look at your to-do list that you started in Chapter 4. Expand it. Add any new items you think of that feel to you like they belong on the list.
- Do at least two tasks that you've been putting off. Any two. Check them off when you complete them.

Week One: Developing Your Food Plan

- Eat three times a day. Meals should have beginnings and endings. No more standing in front of the fridge, mindlessly sampling whatever is there. In addition, two small snacks constructed from the "A" list is fine
- Eat at least *one food* from the "A" list on a daily basis.

This week is about keeping records, and about the beginning of mindfulness. It's about noticing things. You're not going to have to make too many actual changes, but I am going to ask you to begin being more conscious of what you're actually doing. Remember that in order to make changes we have to first know what we're dealing with, and that's the main focus of this week's assignment. Be rigorous with that journal. If anything interesting pops up for you, put it down.

Week One: Exercise

The Shape Up program consists of two simple components: walking and strength training. The strength training exercises will be added in week two. For week one, however, all you have to do is the following:

• Walk ten minutes, three times this week.

These need to be "mindful" walks—in other words, set the time aside, and go for it. I don't care how fast or slow you go. Remember that it's not important how much you do right now. What we're going for is *habit development*. The *fact* that you *do* it is far more important right now than the *amount* you do, a point I covered much more fully in Chapter 7. So do those ten minutes. At least three times during the week.

(If exercise is already a part of your life, go to the appendix, choose the level that seems most appropriate to your current state of fitness and do the corresponding assignments for the next eight weeks. If you're not sure which level you belong in, pick the easier one. I want you to set this up to be a win. This is not the time to overachieve. Believe me, it will build up by the time we're done, so start as easily as you like.)

Week One: Self-Assessment Questionnaire

Answer these three questions in your journal:

1. What are your primary goals in life?
2. Where would you like to be, personally and professionally, in five years? In ten years?
3. What are the top five things standing in the way of you achieving those goals?

Finally, don't forget to re-read the contract as often as necessary. (For most people, that's going to be every day!)

Week Two

Week Two: Journal

• Keep writing! If you don't feel like it, jot down "I don't feel like writing today." Just stay in communication with your journal. See if you can begin to notice connections between what you eat and how you feel. This works in both directions—how you eat may influence how you feel (energy, mood, etc.) and, equally important, how you *feel* may influence how you eat. Start to connect the dots.

Week Two: To-Do List

• Do at least *two more things* from the task completion list. Since you're adding stuff to it all the time, you shouldn't be running out of things to do.

Week Two: Developing Your Food Plan

• Eliminate *one food* from the "B" list.
• Add *two foods* from the "A" list.

Week Two: Exercise

• Increase walking program to five days a week, 10 minutes per day.
• Twice a week, after doing your walk, you're going to perform the following exercise. These two days will be called your "weight training" days, and we'll be adding exercises to the routine as we progress. For now, on those two days, perform the following exercise:

CRUNCHES

Lie on the floor with your legs bent, feet flat on the floor and hands clasped behind your head with the elbows touching the ground. Your head should be in position with the body so that you could hold an apple between your chest and your chin (Figure 9.1).

Imagine Velcroing your lower back to the floor. You may feel like you're doing a small pelvic thrust slightly forward to accomplish this. Keep your lower back nice and stable in this position.

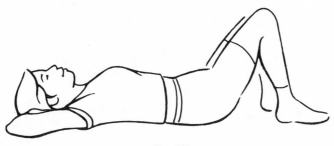

Fig. 9.1

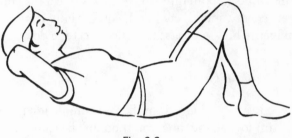

Fig. 9.2

Curl your upper body forward and up holding the highest position (Figure 9.2) for a full second before lowering your upper body back to the ground.

Don't pull on your neck when you come up.

When you lower your upper torso back to the ground, don't return all the way to the "relaxed" position where your weight is supported by the ground, but rather to a point where your upper body is just above the ground and the abs are still contracted.

Remember to keep your elbows all the way back while doing the motion.

Repeat for as many reps as you can manage in good form. The goal is to try for 10–20 repetitions.

Note: I constantly hear from people that they are doing hundreds of crunches. The minute I hear this, I know they're doing them wrong. (I also know there's a good chance they're using momentum and are setting themselves up for a lower back injury.) If you do a crunch properly, it's hard. Most people don't do them correctly. The good news is that when you do them correctly, you don't have to do nearly as many to get results.

Beginners: Remember that if you can only do one or two, that's fine. We'll work up to more, you can bet on it. Don't dwell on what you *can't* do, concentrate on what you *can* do.

Do "Ab Roller" devices work?

Depends on what you mean by "work." Do they help you do ab exercises in good form? Yes. Will they get you a flat tummy that looks like the model on the infomercial in minutes a day? Sorry.

Nearly everyone who wants a flatter tummy really wants to lose fat. What people *really* mean when they point to that midsection and say they want to tone up, is that they want to lose plain old garden variety fat, which for most of us accumulates around our middle. Or our thighs and hips. Or both.

And that's why the magic, "minutes a day" routines are a scam. Because—hear me now—no amount of crunches, no matter how religiously you do them, is going to get rid of fat around your middle. Fat comes off by eating in a way that causes the body to go into its "savings account" of fat and start using it up for energy. It comes off by burning calories through exercise. Lots of it. And it comes off when you increase your metabolic rate by building muscle. And when you stop eating the way you did when you put that fat on in the first place.

So does that mean those ab routines are a waste?

Not on your life.

Your abs are part of your core musculature. They, along with your lower back, are responsible for your posture and your carriage and are essential to a well-toned, fit body. They assist in dozens of movements and exercises. And they help you feel strong and centered.

And if you don't have well-trained, well-developed abs, it won't matter how much fat you lose, you still won't like the way you look when you're thinner. Because to get that rippled effect, there has to be something underneath to ripple.

So. Flat tummy in minutes a day? 'Fraid not. That is, not unless those minutes are accompanied by a rethinking of the eating style that put on the unwanted layer covering those abs in the first place.

To review: Here's what your exercise program is looking like as of now:

Day One	Day Two	Day Three	Day Four	Day Five
walk 10 min.	walk 10 min. crunches	walk 10 min.	walk 10 min. crunches	walk 10 min.

Week Two: Self-Assessment Questionnaire

1. How would you rate your overall level of satisfaction in your day-to-day life?
2. What actions could you take right now to increase the level of personal satisfaction in your day-to-day life?

3. What obstacles, if any, do you see in taking those actions? What's standing in the way of you doing at least one of the actions you listed above *today?*
4. Who could support you most in taking those actions? Who could you count on?
5. Who would *not* support you in taking those actions? Why?
6. Finally, don't forget to re-read the contract as often as necessary. (For most people, that's going to be every day!)

NUTRITIONAL CONTROVERSIES, NUTRITIONAL HERESIES

The formulation of a problem is
far more essential than its solution.

—ALBERT EINSTEIN

There's an old story about a Zen master and a new student who came to him to learn about Zen. The master asked the new student, "Would you like a cup of tea?" Flattered, the student accepted, and held out his cup. The master began to pour the tea until the cup was full. Then, to the student's astonishment, the master kept pouring. The cup overflowed, and the tea spilled out onto the floor, yet the master kept pouring, showing no signs that he had noticed what was happening. Confused and embarrassed, the student didn't know what to do or say. Did he risk offending the master by pointing out the minor flood that was beginning to surround the student's shoes, or did he just ignore it? As the tea continued to pour onto the floor, the student finally blurted out, "But master, the cup is already full!" "Yes," said the master calmly, "and that cup is like your mind. Your mind is like a vessel. You cannot learn Zen until you empty your mind of everything that you came in here with. Only then, when your vessel is open and empty, can I help you fill it with wisdom."

While no Eastern mystic, I've had experience in my own life with the type of frustration experienced by the Zen master. Many years ago, I taught jazz piano for a living. The interesting thing about teaching piano to beginners is that they rarely come in with any preconceived notions. You tell them to hold their wrists a certain way—they do it. Tell them to move their thumbs under the wrist in a fluid motion to better make contact with the keys—they do it. Give them a basic set of chords on which to practice improvisation, and they eagerly take on the task. Here's what they *don't* do: They *don't* come in and say, "But I read that Herbie Hancock does it differently, how come we're not doing it like *he* does it?" or "There was a news item on Channel 7 last night saying that the Russian school bends the wrist at a *lower* height. Shouldn't we be practicing like that?" They just do what you tell them. In a Zen sense, they come to class with an empty cup.

Jazz piano is one thing. Nutrition, however, is another matter entirely. Teaching nutritional information is like pouring tea into an already overflowing cup. In no other field (except perhaps politics, which nutrition resembles far more than most people realize) does everyone have an opinion; not only an opinion, in fact, but a *strongly held* opinion. It's impossible to talk to the average person about what she should be eating, or how she could best manage her weight, or what a healthy diet consists of without encountering a litany of comments referring to what she's read, heard, seen on television, been told by a friend or experienced herself. The media saturates us with information, every television news show has a science reporter who reports on nutrition, every women's magazine has a feature article on dieting in nearly every issue, the Internet has exploded with fitness and diet sites, and two-thirds of America has been, at one time or another, on a diet. In this atmosphere of informational and experiential glut, virtually no one's cup is empty.

Worse, everyone thinks they know what they should be doing, and thinks further that their only problem is not doing it. Much of the time what someone *thinks* they ought to be doing to lose weight is the exact opposite of what they *really* should be doing. I've seen women with more than 100 pounds to lose religiously trying to avoid any fat in their diet when adding some fat (and reducing some carbohydrate) might be exactly what they needed. I've seen people following vegetarian diets not for any ethical or moral reasons, which is a separate issue entirely, but because they mistakenly believe that being vegetarian automatically confers a healthy status on their diet and will help them lose weight. I've seen hundreds of people who are completely confused as to why they're not losing weight when all they eat is "good" stuff like rice cakes and popcorn and salad. They come to me to help them develop a better way to follow a game plan that *should never have been the game plan in the first place.* My job—though at first most clients don't recognize it—is not to tell them how to properly execute what's basically a faulty strategy; rather, it's to *teach them to rethink the strategy altogether.* The wrong strategy, no matter how artfully applied, never wins the game.

One of Jonny's parables:

A gardener is given the assignment to go out and landscape his new boss's estate. Eager to show what a good job he can do, he organizes his employees and together they go out to the site, mow the lawn flawlessly, trim the hedges, replant the flowers, and set up a beautiful Kabuki rock garden right at the entrance to the house. Stunning work, no question about it.

At the end of the day, the boss is driven to the estate. "So what do you think?" asks the gardener, proudly.

Long pause.

"Gorgeous work," says the boss . . .

". . . *but it's not my house.*"

I think of this marvelous story every time I'm asked a question about the best way to cut calories, or the best place to find low-fat recipes, or the best way to follow the food pyramid. Since they're not the best questions to ask in the first place, answering them is like efficiently landscaping the wrong estate.

To Get Good Information, You Have to Ask the Right Questions

There is no shortage of good information about dieting and exercise. What we *do* have is a shortage of good questions. See, most questions contain unstated assumptions that completely skew the nature of the answer (and the usefulness of the information you wind up getting). Most diet books jump right in and try to answer those commonly asked questions without ever questioning the assumptions the questions are based on. Here's an example: Let's say I'm an explorer going off into the New World around the time of Columbus. I consult with the top navigational experts of the day in hopes that they can answer the following question: *What's the best route to take to avoid falling off the edge of the world?* You can see immediately that the nature of the question itself forces a kind of answer that ultimately won't be very useful. Why? *Because both the question and the answer are based on the premise that the world is flat!*

See if you can find the underlying assumptions in the following questions: How do I lower my cholesterol? How can I reduce the fat in my diet? How many calories do I burn on the exercise bike? How many calories should I eat? How can I get 1,500 mg a day of calcium?

The above questions may seem eminently reasonable to you because the assumptions that underlie them are so widely accepted as truth. But, as we'll see, lowering cholesterol by itself doesn't necessarily lower risk for heart disease. Not everyone needs to be on a low-fat diet (and the *kind* of fat you eat is way more important than the *amount*). How many calories you burn during a given exercise session may not be the most important factor in losing weight (building muscle is far more important). And there's a lot more to bone health than just calcium intake (such as reducing the calcium robbers in our diet, like sugar, and getting the proper amounts of supporting minerals, like magnesium).

So to get good information—and by "good" I mean useful to *you*—you need to begin to ask the right questions. I used to do the following demonstration with my personal training students. I'd ask them how they would answer a client who just asked them, "What's the best exercise for the chest?" Several hands would go up, each suggesting a different exercise and making a case for why it was "the best." I'd listen to their answers, and then tell them that if I were the client I'd fire them. Can you guess why? *Because the question can't be answered properly without first asking another question: "For whom and for what purpose?"* The best exercise for the chest is going to be very different if you're a professional bodybuilder one week away from a big contest, or if you're Mrs. Jones who has never worked out before and wants to build enough upper body strength to open a jar! If you don't establish who it is you're talking about, any answer to the question is not only premature, but downright useless.

What would you think about a doctor who answered the question, "What's the best medicine?" without asking a few questions of his own? Like, "Best medicine for *what*? A cold? Arthritis? Diabetes? HIV? A sinus infection?" What stockbroker worth his commission would answer the question, "What's the best stock to buy?" without first questioning the client about her financial needs, tolerance for risk, liquidity and the like?

As I've said before, a program that teaches you what to do but doesn't help you to actually *do* it is not very useful. *However, a program that answers the wrong questions is not very useful either.* The Shape Up program is going to start you off with the right information—or at least show you how to find it for yourself—so that you can spend the rest of our time together developing effective strategies for putting that information into action.

So in the spirit of clearing a path toward better information, let's begin by emptying our teacups of one of the biggest misconceptions in old-fashioned, orthodox nutrition: the food pyramid.

Why the Food Pyramid Is Bad for Your Health

It is a very myopic medical science that works backward from the morgue rather than forward from the cradle.

—*E. A. HOOTON, FROM* AN ANTHROPOLOGIST LOOKS AT MEDICINE

I'm often asked, "What's wrong with the food pyramid?"

Well, off the record, just between us, I usually answer that question with one word: *everything.*

The USDA food pyramid, the current version of which was published in 1992, is "committee-think," and in this case the committee is composed of representatives from the food industry plus the most entrenched and conservative factors of academic nutrition and medicine. As Robert Crayhon says, "It is a product of both expert lobbying and mediocre science." Amen. It's the government's second try at coming up with a general template that they recommend for everyone (anyone remember the four food groups?), and it undoubtedly won't be their last. *You,* however, don't have to wait till they finally figure out what's wrong with it to throw it out.

Here are the top eight things that are wrong with the USDA food pyramid.

1. The food pyramid is based on the demonstrably false assumption that everyone needs the same foods and that there is one healthy diet that works for everyone. You've already learned to raise an eyebrow when you hear that bit of conventional wisdom, which is neither conventional nor wise, and hopefully you'll be raising that eyebrow even higher by the time you finish the program. Furthermore, the diet the committee chose to anoint as the one and only healthy way to eat is the familiar low-fat, high-carbohydrate diet that has caused such problems for virtually everyone for whom weight has been a lifelong struggle. The bottom line: One size *doesn't* fit all, and even if it did, it probably wouldn't be this size.

2. The food pyramid encourages you to think that fats are the "bad guy." If there's one concept that's been wholesaled to us as a nation, it's the idea that it's healthy to reduce fat intake to as low as possible. Making a case *against* this concept often causes people to look at you as if you just said that aliens are speaking to you through the fillings in your teeth, but nonetheless, the concept of wholesale fat avoidance is utterly wrong-headed. There are different kinds of fats, and many of them are downright necessary for good health. Fats are the raw materials of many substances that are critical for human health, including eicosanoids, hormones and, yes, cholesterol (without which you couldn't live).

Interestingly, *eating* some fats may even help you *lose* fat. Ann Louise Gittleman, formerly the nutrition director for the ultra-low-fat Pritikin Center and a "reformed" low-fat advocate, reports that she now adds essential fatty acids to the diets of many previously "fat-free" women who were stuck at a weight plateau and that the addition of these healthy fats has jump-started their weight loss.

The food pyramid makes no distinction among the different kinds of fats, just as it doesn't distinguish among the different kinds of carbohydrates (see No. 4). Fact is, the fats found in cold-water fish, nuts, avocados, and olive oil are among the most healthful substances you can possibly eat. Even some members of the universally demonized saturated fat group may have health benefits—lauric acid, for example, found in butter and coconut, is antiviral, and some traditional fats like butter (far, far better for you than margarine) are an unsurpassed source of vitamin A.

3. The food pyramid lumps fats and sugars together.   The food pyramid demonizes both fats and sugars and tells you to eat both sparingly. As you are discovering, fats and sugars are very different animals and have very different effects on the body. Some fats should be increased (see above); nearly all sugars should be *decreased* as much as possible.

Basic sugar is not only non-nutritive, it's *anti*-nutritive. Here's why: When sugar is found in real life foods and plants, like sugar cane, for example, it contains the vitamins, minerals, and enzymes needed for its complete digestion. When it is found in your sugar bowl it contains none of these and actually has to "borrow" from your body's stores of these nutrients in order to process it. That's why many nutritionists consider sugar to be an immune system depressor. It literally steals from the nutrient stores your body needs to stay healthy in order to metabolize it.

Furthermore, there's a school of thought that believes many of us are "sugar sensitive," meaning we react very badly to sugar of any kind. Sugar has demonstrated abilities to modulate pain thresholds and acts in your brain much like an endorphin. For this reason, the concept of sugar addiction, particularly for people with susceptible brain chemistry, is gaining a lot of currency in integrative and alternative medicine and nutritional circles (although you'll rarely hear anything about it from conservatively trained doctors or dietitians). And if you think the insane amount of sugar we are now routinely feeding our kids isn't affecting more than their waistlines, think again. A recent study at California State University manipulated the diets of kids in 803 schools and nine juvenile correctional facilities. They gave them, among other things, more fruits and vegetables and less fat and sugar. The results were astonishing. Grades rose 16 percent, and, even more telling, *the number classified as learning-disabled fell by almost half.* Without going too far afield here, let me just say this: Attention deficit disorder is not a

Ritalin deficiency. We ignore the sugar and nutrition connection at our own peril.

According to most estimates, we're now taking in an unprecedented 20 percent of our calories from sugar, and that number is growing every day. These sugars are most often in the form of convenience and packaged foods. Fat-free foods are some of the worst offenders. Remember our old friend insulin? Well, nothing raises it like sugar, and as we've seen, consistently high levels of insulin make it virtually impossible to lose weight, not to mention making it a lot more probable that you will be a lot less healthy. Which leads us to the million dollar question: Why does the food industry and medical establishment continue to tell us that the best way to lose weight is to eat the very foods that raise insulin levels?

4. The food pyramid makes no distinctions among types of carbohydrates. The pyramid provides no inherent way of distinguishing junk carbohydrates from the real deal: One serving of slow-cooking whole-grain oatmeal would be equal to the same amount of the latest Choco-Chipo-Krunchy-Krispy cold cereal. That's like telling everyone to buy a car and forgetting to tell them the difference between Yugos and Mercedes.

Cauliflower and Twinkies are both carbohydrates, just as DHA and margarine are both fats. There is a huge difference between carbohydrates from vegetables and low-sugar high-fiber fruits like berries and the junk carbohydrates that fill most of our plates. The Shape Up plan does *not* recommend "no carbohydrates"—it recommends no *junk* carbohydrates. There's a big difference.

5. The base of the food pyramid consists of foods that will cause many people to gain weight. Most commercial pastas, breads and cereals are nothing more than highly refined, processed foods without any fiber and with most of the nutrients missing, even though the food industry throws a few back in after the fact in a weak attempt to correct the damage. These foods raise blood sugar quickly, leading to a surge of insulin and setting in motion a whole roller coaster of events that ultimately result in both weight gain and poor health. The orthodox nutrition establishment tries to weasel out of this predicament by giving lip service to whole grains, which are definitely an improvement over the refined ones, but the problem is this: Most Americans have never seen a whole grain. The commercial products on the market, despite an effort to market to the idea that "brown is better," are usually little more than refined grains with a bit of whole wheat thrown in, or sometimes just some coloring. Remember that just because something started life as a whole grain doesn't automatically mean that you're getting any health benefits from it by the time it's been turned into commercial bread. The whole process of making flour out of any whole grain involves so much pulverization, processing, and heating that very few nutrients are left by the time it winds up on your plate.

Furthermore, many nutritionists and researchers are now questioning our overconsumption of grains *in general*. It's far from clear that grains ought to make up the bulk of our diet. Wheat, for example, is one of the ten most common allergens, and in susceptible people can cause bloating and a host of other more serious symptoms often unattributed to the amount of wheat (or other grains) they are consuming. Remember that grains are a pretty "late comer" from an evolutionary, Paleolithic perspective. As Loren Cordain points out in *Cereal Grains: Humanity's Double Edged Sword*, it's pretty unlikely that the planet will be able to survive without adapting to grains as a food source—but that doesn't mean that you as an individual with other options available need to rely on them nearly as heavily as the food pyramid folks think you should. The brilliant researcher Dr. C. Leigh Broadhurst once said to me that if she had to pick one strategy to recommend to chronically overweight people it would be to cut out wheat. At the very least, it's something to think about.

So why in the world do wheat and grain products get the lion's share of the food pyramid? Well, if I went to the XYZ Dog Chow company and asked them to make a food pyramid for dogs, what do you think would be on it? Do you need a second guess? I've got news for you: Left to their own devices in the wild, dogs don't eat XYZ Dog Chow. They eat what their canine ancestors have eaten for as long as they've been on the planet. Like us, their basic plumbing hasn't changed. Preparing food that our domesticated best friends naturally prefer may not be as easy as opening a can or ripping open an easy-pour bag, but that is what they were built to eat nonetheless. I'm not saying there's anything wrong with letting the XYZ Dog Chow companies of the world help us out here, but I am saying it's a little dangerous when you let them, under the guise of scientific objectivity, be responsible for teaching us dog nutrition.

Think that doesn't happen here? Take this pop quiz: What is the number one source for nutritional information in the United States?

The dairy industry. Which leads us nicely to our next questionable assumption:

6. **The food pyramid assumes everyone should have dairy.** Fully more than half the world's population is lactose intolerant (75 percent in the case of African Americans), which may cause bloating, abdominal pain and diarrhea after milk is consumed. So it's hard to understand the food pyramid recommendation that everyone should consume two to three servings of dairy a day until you recall that the dairy industry is the number one source of nutritional information in this country. Being hammered with slogans like "You never outgrow your need for milk" and cute ads featuring gorgeous models with milk moustaches does not change the fact that milk is hardly a healthy nor necessary food for adults. Naturally fermented dairy products like yogurt[1] are a different story and are often tolerated well even by people who don't tolerate milk. And certain cheeses, like natural Swiss, are a far better source of calcium than milk in any case.

The bottom line: Dairy isn't for everyone, and all dairy isn't created equal.

7. **The food pyramid is aimed at the "average person."** There is no such thing as the average person. Think about it: In what way are *you* average? It's demonstrably true that people of different ages, sexes, stress levels, activity levels, genetics, and metabolic types have different nutritional needs—sometimes dramatically so. Even *you* at different points in your life have substantially different needs. How is it possible for the same old tired nutritional formula to be perfect for an active eighteen-year-old, a stressed out college student, an expectant mother, an active thirty-eight-year-old mother of two, a menopausal CEO, and a senior citizen bicycling around the country? The answer: It's not.

8. **The food pyramid makes no allowances for seasonal changes in eating habits.** One of the many differences between our Paleolithic, hunter-gatherer forebears and us is that they didn't have supermarkets. Through the modern miracles of manufacturing, processing, preserving, and transporting, the food industry has made it possible for us to have any kind of food, any time of year, anywhere in the world. This is quite out of sync with our long-buried ancestral impulses to go out into the woods and gather and hunt whatever is available at a particular time of year. One of the few principles of macrobiotic eating with which I agree is the one that suggests you eat what is grown locally and in season. Stuff changes. Many people are more active in the warm weather and more sedentary in the cold. This in turn affects all kinds of things, including mood, serotonin production, and even insulin sensitivity (vitamin D-3, which you get from

sun exposure, has an effect on glucose metabolism). Your environment is not static and neither are you, and it might just be a good idea to let your eating habits mirror that pulse. Fruits, for example, cool and hydrate the body, something we need far more of in the summer months than we do in the winter. Some rotation of foods may also be advisable from a food sensitivity point of view. The "all-pyramid, all-the-time" approach makes no allowance for this.

I'll go on record as saying that I think the Shape Up plan for health and weight loss is a far healthier and more flexible set of guidelines to use than the USDA food pyramid. Here's the recipe:

Protein from high-quality sources, like eggs, whey protein powder, lean organic meats, free range poultry, and uncontaminated fish, tons and tons of vegetables, low-sugar, high-fiber fruits like berries, and fat from the best sources on the planet like fish, nuts, avocados, extra-virgin cold-pressed olive oil, flaxseed, coconut, and occasionally butter. Some raw foods or vegetable juices every day. Small amounts of "good guy" starches like sweet potatoes, oatmeal, and maybe lentils or beans. Add to the menu naturally fermented products like miso, tempeh, yogurt, and kefir. If you like, have some cheese, especially soft ones, or ones made from raw milk. The exact mix, proportions and amounts to be determined by each individual.

That basic buffet is one on which you can live healthily for the rest of your life.

A Word About Fat

Let's talk a little about fat.

Many nutritionists believe that essential fatty acid deficiency is one of the major—if not *the* major—problem in the American diet. There are two fatty acids that are considered essential—that is, they can't be made by the body and therefore must be obtained from the diet. The technical names for these fats are *linoleic acid* and *alpha-linolenic acid*. The former is a member of a subgroup called "omega-6s" and the latter belongs to a sub-group called "omega-3s." Our Paleolithic ancestors, and most hunter-gatherer societies, consumed these in a healthy ratio of somewhere between 1:1 and 4:1, which is what most nutritionists consider the proper balance. *The ratio in the modern diet is somewhere around 20:1.* This imbalance is considered by many people in my neck of the woods to be one of the great health issues of our time. Furthermore, the omega-6s are a pretty big family, and the ones that we are so overconsuming are hardly the best of the lot—many are coming from refined vegetable oils (the cooking oils on your grocer's shelf that proudly proclaim "no choles-terol"!). These oils have a great shelf life, but at a cost—the cost in this case is that in order to stay on the shelf without going rancid, they must have virtually all of their antioxidants (like vitamin E) and other nutrients stripped from them. Even Barry Sears, an advocate of the use of soy, decries the use of soybean oil—the most commonly used vegetable oil—because its abundance of omega-6 fatty acids adds fuel to the fire of this serious nutritional imbalance. The lack of balance in our diet between the two families of fats can be corrected only by consuming much more of the omega-3 family (found in fish) and much less of the omega-6 (refined vegetable oils and the like).

Many nutritionists continue to recommend flaxseed oil because it is a good source of the essential omega-3 fatty acid mentioned above, alpha-linolenic acid (ALA). While it's true that flax meal has healthful properties (including fiber) and the flax oil does contain ALA, the main reason we recommended flax was because ALA is the *raw material* from which the body makes the even *more* important members of the omega-3 family.

Here's how it works: The term "fat" as we commonly use it actually refers to a collection of smaller units called fatty acids. A *fatty acid* is itself made up of even smaller units—a chain of carbon atoms joined together by chemical bonds. Each carbon atom has the chemical equivalent of four hands, four "parking spots" where it can bond with other atoms. In a fatty acid, two of these hands are reserved for hydrogen atoms; one hand attaches to the next carbon molecule in the chain, and the last hand attaches to the carbon molecule behind it.

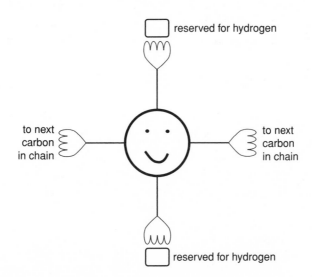

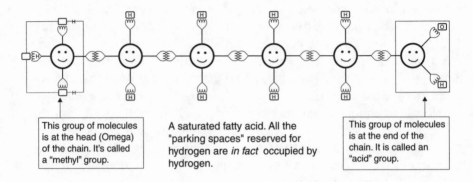

This group of molecules is at the head (Omega) of the chain. It's called a "methyl" group.

A saturated fatty acid. All the "parking spaces" reserved for hydrogen are *in fact* occupied by hydrogen.

This group of molecules is at the end of the chain. It is called an "acid" group.

If both the hands reserved for hydrogen are in fact *occupied* by hydrogen, that carbon is said to be *saturated*—its dance card is filled. If all the carbons *in the entire chain* of carbons have their "hydrogen hands" filled with hydrogen, that whole fatty acid is considered saturated; when most of the fatty acids that make up what we call a fat are built according to this architecture, we classify the fat itself as a "*saturated fat.*"

Sometimes only *one* hydrogen atom attaches to the four-handed carbon atom instead of two—when this occurs, the *other* hand normally "reserved" for hydrogen goes instead to strengthening the bond to the next carbon in the line, kind of like a "double handshake."

This stronger chemical connection between two carbon atoms in the link is called, understandably, a "double bond," and as soon as there's at least one of these in the chain, the fatty acid is no longer considered saturated (because at least *one* of the hydrogen "parking spaces" isn't being occupied by hydrogen). When only *one* such double bond exists in a

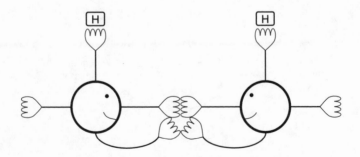

This location is no longer "saturated" with hydroden because two adjacent carbons are doing a "double handshake" instead of each holding a hydrogen atom.

A "monounsaturated" fatty acid. It is monounsaturated because there is only one "double handshake," and thus only one pair of carbons (between 9–10) which aren't saturated with hydrogen. This particular fatty acid has 18 carbons, is called "oleic acid" and is plentiful in olive oil.

whole chain of carbons, the fatty acid is considered a member of the "monounsaturated" family; when *more than one* double bond occurs in the chain, it's called "polyunsaturated." (In fact, all fats are really *collections* of *saturated* fatty acids, *polyunsaturated* fatty acids and *monounsaturated* fatty acids, but we tend to name the fat itself by the type of fatty acid that *predominates* in the mix. Thus extra-virgin, cold-pressed olive oil is commonly referred to as a "monounsaturated fat" because this is the fatty acid family that predominates in olive oil, but in fact olive oil—like all fats and oils—contains all three fatty acid families.)

You might think from the above discussion that there are only three ways for carbons to arrange themselves in a chain, but unfortunately it's not that simple. While all fatty acids do in fact arrange themselves into one of three *categories*—saturated, monounsaturated and polyunsaturated— these categories are like cities. Each city can be further broken down into neighborhoods, and each neighborhood has block associations, and each block association is made up of many individual members. As in any collection of individuals, some members of the group are superstars and make invaluable contributions to the health and robustness of the community—in this case the body—while some individuals are problem citizens. In the case of fatty acids, there are two superstars, which, among other things, contribute to brain health, help fight depression, are anti-inflammatory, improve heart health and can reduce blood pressure. Both are made up of long chains of carbons (which is why they are known as the "long-chain fatty acids"), both are members of the polyunsaturated family and both have their first "double bond" at the third carbon position in the chain (which is why they are also members of a subgroup known as "omega-3" fatty acids). These two superstars have the imposing names of eicosapentaenoic acid (weighing in with twenty carbons in its chain and five double bonds along the route) and docosahexaenoic acid (twenty-two carbons in its chains and six double bonds along the route). Fortunately these fatty acids are known by their nicknames, EPA (for eicosapentaenoic acid) and DHA (for docosahexaenoic acid).

And we're not eating nearly enough of either one.

Now, in the best of all possible worlds, the body will *make* these two superstar fatty acids from the raw material of our old friend the essential fatty acid alpha-linolenic acid. And that's one of the selling points of flaxseed oil—give the body the raw materials and it will build what it needs.

Except it doesn't always happen that way.

The route from alpha-linolenic acid—weighing in with eighteen carbons in the chain, three double bonds along the route—to the longer chain EPA and DHA is a long and arduous journey, and the body does not always perform this transformation successfully. Therefore, even if you take flaxseed oil as a supplement, it's no guarantee that you will be getting enough of these superstar fatty acids that still have to be made from the raw materials in the flaxseed oil. Even though I still recommend using flaxseed oil as an oil (never for cooking, however) and putting flax meal into drinks and recipes, I no longer recommend it as a way of ensuring that you're getting enough EPA and DHA. I now prefer that my clients take the real deal—fish oil, which is ready-made EPA and DHA. That way we don't have to worry about all the things that could break down on that long, arduous path of *desaturation* and *elongation* that needs to take place in the body in order to morph alpha-linolenic acid into EPA and DHA. Why not just take the DHA and EPA directly and not have to worry about everything that could go wrong along the way? That seems to me a much better strategy than giving the body the raw materials and just hoping for the best.

And what's the best source of these vitally important fatty acids?

Well, there was a reason your grandmother told you to take cod liver oil, and there was a reason she said that fish was "brain food." It's because fish (or fish oil) is the best way to get these two superstar fatty acids. (DHA, in particular, makes up a large percentage of the fat in your brain, and I can think of almost no supplement more important for a nursing mother to take.)

The fat story doesn't end with this, however. In an effort to market to a population frightened to death of saturated fat, the food industry has filled our foods with a particularly dangerous kind of fatty acid called "trans-fatty acids." These human-made fats, which are in just about every baked and packaged food product imaginable and are rampant in margarine, are damaged fats that have had hydrogen force-fed into them to make them more stable, changing their configuration from the healthy "cis" form to the quite unhealthy "trans" form. Technically they're not saturated fats, but they're actually a lot worse. If the label says "hydrogenated" or "partially hydrogenated" anything, you know it contains trans-fats. I'm far more concerned about our intake of these babies than I am of almost any other kind of fat. Fried foods—especially in commercial fast-food restaurants that use cheap oils and then reheat them time and again—are a virtual breeding ground for trans-fats. Think about that next time you see a commercial for super-sized fries.

Fats are needed to make cell membranes, among other things. These membranes need to have just the right combination of strength and flexibility. Saturated fats provide the strength and stability; omega-3s provide the flexibility that allow important nutrients to get in and out of the cells. Trans-fatty acids, and other damaged fats, are like rotten wood. If you have to build a house in the forest for shelter, and there's absolutely nothing else around, you'll use the rotting lumber, but the house ain't gonna make it to *Architectural Digest*. These trans-fatty acids get into our cell membranes and do all kinds of mischief. They should be avoided like the bubonic plague. But to put them in the same category as superstars like EPA and DHA—remember, the food pyramid makes no distinctions here—is like lumping a broken-down, rat-infested tenement apartment with a palatial estate on the ocean because both are technically "shelter."

There *is* some reason to avoid very fatty meats, however, but it's not the reason commonly given. Toxins are stored in fat. The fat of our factory farmed animals, fed an unnatural (for them) diet of grains instead of grass and shot full of hormones and antibiotics, is now a toxic waste dump for stuff you don't want to have in your body. For that reason alone, unless you can get your hands on free-range, drug-free game, it's probably a good idea to keep your intake of animal fat low and to buy the best and leanest cuts of meat you can afford. Organically raised if at all possible.

Many societies consume much more fat than the food pyramid recommends—the Mediterraneans, for example, or the Inuit of Greenland—yet have far less heart disease than we do. The problem is not fat per se, obviously, but the *kind* of fat. And it's hard to ignore the fact that while the fat-free food industry experienced a growth spurt, so did obesity rates. Fat is not the enemy here—ignorance is.

Bottom line: Eat more of the good fats from fish like salmon, mackerel and sardines, nuts, avocados, olives, extra virgin cold-pressed olive oil, flaxseed, coconut, and even reasonable amounts of some traditional fat, like fresh creamy butter. Eat less or none of the bad fats, like refined and processed vegetable oils, margarine, any packaged baked good that says "hydrogenated" or "partially hydrogenated" in the ingredients list, and *especially* anything that's been fried, particularly in fast-food restaurants.

Sugar: The Bad and the Ugly

Tattoo this in your brain: Sugar turns to fat.

But first, a little background and a quiz.

Percentage of Americans who are overweight: 54 percent (in 1999) and rising, up from 33 percent (in 1991) and 25 percent in 1976. At least 20 percent are considered obese. Quick, take a guess as to why.

Think it's calories? Well, maybe—they went up a little bit but not enough to explain all of it, and definitely not enough to account for the epidemic increase in type II diabetes. Try again.

Must be eating more fat, right? Sorry. During the same period fat consumption dropped about 5 percent, from around 41 percent of the diet to 37 percent.

Give up?

Well, at the risk of oversimplifying a complex issue, here's my guess: sugar. In 1970, the average American ate about 121 pounds of the stuff in a typical year. In 1992, it was up to 142 pounds (recent data suggest it's moving up into the 145-pound range). And it's everywhere, folks. Hiding out in foods under disguises like brown rice syrup, fruit juice concentrate, high-fructose corn syrup, confectioners sugar, corn syrup, date sugar, maltodextrin, maltose, mannitol, sorbitol, xylitol, and turbinado sugar, just to name a few.

Addictions? Well, you tell me. Ask smokers to describe what it's like when they can't have a smoke they crave, and then tell me what food craving that sounds like to you. I'll betcha a buck it's not broccoli.

Houston, we got a biiiiiiggggg problem here.

In the mania for low-fat diets and fat-free foods, Americans started replacing that dreaded fat with carbohydrates. The buzz was that since most protein sources were also loaded with fat, they should be limited as well. What was left to eat? Well, you do the math. If you can't eat fat and you have to limit protein, all that's left is—carbohydrates! Unfortunately, most of the carbohydrates that we turned to were junky, processed, refined food products, many—like pasta and bagels—marketed as healthy because they didn't contain fat.

It gets worse.

All those "healthy" foods like cereal and bread that are at the bottom of the USDA food pyramid are nothing more than refined, processed, fiberless commercial products that usually convert to sugar in your body, almost as fast as the real thing, causing blood sugar surges and eventuallychronically elevated insulin levels. As anyone who's read a nutrition book in the last ten years knows, this is not a good thing. The blood sugar roller coaster sets you up for the vicious cycle of hunger, cravings, weight gain, loss of energy, more cravings, the inability to lose fat, moodiness and worse. You, my friend, are in "sugar hell."

Folks, if you want to do something really good for yourself, get the sugar out.

I know, I know. Easier said than done, right?

So here are some tips to start with. Understand that this is a long and winding road, and few people are going to be able to do it perfectly, let alone the first time out. But if you can begin to raise your consciousness about sugar and junk carbohydrates, and begin reducing their contribution to your diet, you will be taking measurable steps toward improving both your health and your weight. Trust me.

1. **Be a sugar zealot.** Look on the label under "Total Carbohydrates" and, under that, "Sugars." Look for relatively low numbers. FYI: 4 grams of sugar equals 1 teaspoon. Think of that the next time you eat a cereal that has 25 grams of sugar per tiny serving size! And while we're on the subject of cereals . . .

2. **Read labels.** Look under fiber. The number should be as high as possible. I like Dr. Bob Arnot's "five and five" rule for cereals: *less* than 5 grams of sugar, 5 or *more* of fiber. Few cereals make the cut, but do the best you can.

3. **Avoid fat-free foods.** They're loaded with either or both of two things: artificial stuff or sugar. Neither is good for you, and the calories are empty.

4. **Avoid pure sugar hits like fruit juice.** Begin to gravitate more toward pure water, herbal teas and flavored non-caloric seltzers (without artificial sweeteners!). Flavor the water with lemon if you like. If you need a transitional beverage, use water with just a little fruit juice for flavor. Or mix a small amount of unsweetened cranberry juice with a large amount of water and get even more benefits.

5. **Mix and match.** You can lessen the sugar load of a food like pasta, if you're not ready to give it up entirely, by adding some meat or turkey or a heaping portion of colorful vegetables or both. Protein, fat and

fiber all slow the entrance of sugar into the digestive system. The trick is to use a really small portion of the pasta in the first place.

6. **Try something else.** When you have a sugar craving, see if you can satisfy it with something less likely to produce a cascade of unpleasant blood sugar events, something like an apple with some peanut butter, or a celery stick with crunchy almond butter. Sometimes spicy foods like a pickle will help defuse the sweet craving.

7. **Take your chromium picolinate.** Minimum 200 mcg a day, preferably more (400 mcg on the Shape Up supplement plans). Chromium helps insulin do its job—it's helpful for blood sugar management, and it's virtually impossible to get enough from your diet.

8. **Try L-glutamine.** For strong sugar cravings, the amino acid L-glutamine has been found helpful by many people. Stir a couple of spoonfuls in some water, drink, and wait for twenty minutes.

9. **Be proactive.** Small meals throughout the day help keep blood sugar even, and may help keep cravings at bay. Eat some protein at every meal, and keep the fiber as high as you can. And don't be afraid of the good fats like extra-virgin cold-pressed olive oil, nuts, and even some fresh creamy butter. Just don't go crazy.

Finally . . .

1. Know that this is a process not an event. It may take some time. Know also that if you can stick it out, cravings do subside.

Fake Sugar

Years ago when I was growing up, my father used to regularly repeat the following mantra of parental wisdom, common among parents of baby boomers like myself: "There are two things you never discuss in public," he'd say. "Religion and politics."

The reasoning in that pre-*Oprah* time was that bringing up either of these two subjects in conversation could virtually guarantee a heated (and ultimately unpleasant) discussion, possibly destroy friendships and, at the very least, ruin an evening.

Well, religion and politics are no longer forbidden topics for friendly discourse, but among nutrition experts there are still a few subjects that pretty much assure the kind of messy passion considered so gauche in my parents' time. And making anyone's top-five list for a knock-down, dragout argument is the subject of artificial sweeteners.

Ask members of the food establishment and their apologists and they'll tell you, often with a sneer, that there's no "scientific evidence" that artificial sweeteners—especially aspartame, the ingredient in Equal—cause any problems, except for a small subset of the population with a fairly uncommon metabolic abnormality called phenylketonuria (PKU). Perfectly safe, they sniff. The FDA said so. Drink diet sodas rather than regular ones, and sweeten your coffee all you like. It will help you lose weight because you'll be saving all those calories that you would be otherwise consuming in sugar. All those silly rumors of problems are just that—wild, unsubstantiated rumors with no "scientific" backing. Probably started by Communists. What are they gonna go after next, cell phones?

I'm not so sure.

Aspartame is a molecule made by joining two amino acids together, which makes it a protein fragment. That protein molecule is broken down into two compounds—formaldehyde, a known carcinogen, and methanol (wood alcohol), which is a toxin capable of causing blindness. The FDA decided in its infinite wisdom, with no small amount of pressure from industry, that this wasn't much of an issue since the *amounts* of these two substances generated from the breakdown of aspartame didn't reach toxic levels—hence, the consumer had nothing to worry about. Believe them? Well then you have more faith in your government agencies than I do. I've met more than one person who routinely consumes a dozen cans of diet soda a day, not to mention low-fat or sugar-free desserts (which are filled with the stuff), and even if the FDA were right in thinking that small amounts of the two neurotoxins made from aspartame are "safe," I'm not sure anyone knows the long-term effects of the kind of consumption we're routinely seeing today.

The tiny protein fragment that is aspartame is able to enter the bloodstream and eventually make its way to a place in the brain called the "bare area." Now Nature, in her infinite wisdom, wisely surrounded the brain with a protective shield called the "blood-brain" barrier, meant to guard our delicate brain tissue from any undesirable riffraff that might be cruising around the bloodstream. But in that bare area there's a security gap— a break in the gate—and it's possible for unwanted substances to enter and do some serious mischief. Once inside, they may stimulate the brain in an undesirable way, causing an effect called "excitotoxicity." This is exactly how aspartame, and other molecules like MSG, can theoretically present a serious problem. This point of view has been brilliantly explained and the arguments for it very well elucidated by Russell L. Blaylock, M.D., in his excellent book *Excitotoxins: The Taste That Kills*. It is also a little-reported fact that aspartame accounts for more consumer complaints to the FDA—by some reports as high as 75 percent of complaints—than any other food ingredient.

Moving right along.

In an excellent review article in the January 2000 issue of the *Townsend Newsletter for Doctors and Patients,* Dr. H. J. Roberts chronicles his own extensive experience with the "many serious side effects and medical/public health hazards attributable to aspartame products" (his words, not mine). He believes, based on his database of over 12,000 "aspartame reactors," that aspartame can cause neurological, psychological, endocrine and metabolic problems, that it can cause, aggravate or accelerate migraines, and that in sensitive people it can be downright addictive. Drs. Mary Dan and Michael Eades add that in susceptible people, "Consuming aspartame may result in such symptoms as mood disturbances, sleep disturbances, headaches, dizziness, short-term memory loss, fuzzy thinking and inability to concentrate."

For those who continue to insist, along with the FDA, that there is "no scientific evidence" for a problem, I'd like to say one word to you: cigarettes. The connection between lung cancer and cigarettes was pretty much common knowledge for almost fifteen years before the FDA finally decided there was enough evidence to put a warning on cancer sticks. And the history of nutrition is filled with a huge gap between the discovery of something by pioneers and its widespread acceptance by the powers that be (example: vitamin C as a cure for scurvy). Just some food for thought. Just because something hasn't been definitively proven yet doesn't mean it's not so.

Aside from the health concerns, the funny thing is this: Artificial sweeteners don't even really help you lose weight. They continue to feed your sweet tooth, making you want more sweet stuff, and lessening the chance that you will eventually stop craving sugar. And some research has shown that when people eat what they think is low-fat or low-calorie food, they make up for it by eating more of the wrong things later in the day.

Breaking the sweetener habit may not be so easy, so I recommend that if you must sweeten, do it infrequently—and when you do, use small amounts of the best, richest, darkest honey you can find, or, alternately, a high-quality real (not imitation) maple syrup. You can also use the herb stevia, found in health food stores, but watch the amounts—unless you use just a little, it can have a bitter aftertaste. A relative newcomer to the artificial sweetener line-up that looks promising is sucralose, also known as Splenda, but we'll have to wait and see on this one.

The good side of dumping your artificial sweetener habit is that you will probably drink fewer diet sodas and eat fewer "no-cal" desserts. Even if there were no other benefit to kicking the artificial sweetener habit, that alone would make it worth the effort.

Energy Bars

And what about those energy bars?

Staffers from a well-known glossy magazine recently engineered the following ingenious stunt for the sake of a story: They got some ordinary orange soda, set up a table on a busy city street with little Dixie cups and let the soda get nice and flat. Then they gave out samples of the drink to passersby.

It gets better.

The staffers wore T-shirts that said "Mangoe!" and told the people tasting the drink that it was a new, imported tropical drink that was being test-marketed, and would probably sell for about five bucks a bottle. Then they asked the unsuspecting folks for their comments in the name of market research.

Most people said they loved it.

A few said they'd easily pay five bucks for it.

A few said it was really good but a bit overpriced.

P. T. Barnum would have loved it. But it would be old news to him if he'd been observing the marketing of some health and energy bars.

Take granola bars. I recently plucked one of these babies from a homey-looking wood bin at a well-known coffee chain. The bars were labeled in mock handwritten calligraphy, made to look like they were freshly baked by some nice old lady who then packaged them in her kitchen and drove around in her truck to distribute them to the local general store. The bar itself practically reeked "health food." The salesperson assured me that it was a real healthy snack, being low-fat and all that.

Exhibit A—the list of ingredients: sugar, rolled oats, dextrose, wheat flakes, rice, dried lemon, (sulfited) soybeans, fructose, corn syrup, partially hydrogenated peanut and soybean oil, nonfat milk, almonds, malt, sorbitol, and flavoring.

If you buy that as a health bar, well, there's this great bridge in Brooklyn that I'd like to offer you for sale. . . .

By law, a manufacturer has to list the ingredients on its product by weight. Whatever ingredient is listed first, that's the predominant ingredient in the product. In the case of the above "health" bar, it's a no-brainer:

You're eating sugar and damaged fats in a warm, fuzzy wrapper. But manufacturers are tricky. They know that people are getting wise to how much sugar is in their products, so here's what they do: They put a *small* amount of lots of *different* sugars into the product. That way, no single one of the sugars is the main ingredient by weight; but add them all up, and sugar in all its disguises taken together still outweighs anything else in the recipe.

If you think you aren't eating sugar when you're eating "health" bars, it's time to take another look at those labels.

Real health food is the kind you can grow, pick, pluck, gather, fish, or hunt for.

Choosing "Energy" Bars

Some energy bars are better than others. Given a choice between your average snack machine fare and one of the better "sports" bars made by a reputable company, I'd go with the latter any day. The ones that are about 200 calories with the 40/30/30 formula (PR Ironman, Balance, etc.) would be my preference. Also look for products by Lee Labrada, TwinLabs, and some of the newer high-protein bars, but be aware that a lot of these are marketed to bodybuilders and can be pretty high calorie if you're just using them for a snack.

Note

1. By the way, any resemblance between naturally fermented, healthy yogurts and those fruit-on-the-bottom sugar-loaded desserts at the local mini-mart is purely coincidental.

WEEKS THREE AND FOUR 11

Week Three

Week Three: Journal

Keep writing! What have you noticed in the last two weeks? Have there been any obvious connections between food and mood? How about not-so-obvious connections? What's your energy been like? Have you noticed any resentment about doing these processes? A sense of elation? Empowerment? Discouragement? Sadness? Hopefulness? Hope*less*ness? All of the above? None of the above? Write it down. And here's one further assignment for the week: *Be willing to be wherever you are with this.* As you'll learn throughout this program, despite our best efforts to the contrary, the only place we *can* be is where we *are*. Whatever you're going through, *be* with it. Just keep telling the truth about it, and keep looking.

And when you think there's nothing more to do . . . .

Look some more.

Week Three: To-Do List

The to-do list should begin to look like something in a constant state of revision right about now. You've added some stuff, you've crossed out some stuff, you've probably made some decisions about what belongs and what doesn't belong on the list. I'd like to ask you to try to hold off on judging anything on this list for now. Just keep writing down whatever occurs to you that might be occupying psychic space, whether it's an incomplete term paper, a promised phone call to a friend, a visit, a question you've been meaning to ask someone, a catalogue you've been meaning to send for, an e-mail you've been slow to respond to or a house you've been meaning to buy! Just make sure that this week, and every week, you do *at least* two things on that list and that you check them off when they are complete.

Week Three: Developing Your Food Plan

- Add one more food from the "A" list.
- Eliminate one more food from the "B" list.
- Have protein at each meal. You don't have to weigh and measure, but if you're comfortable doing so, roughly four ounces equals one serving of protein—but don't lose any sleep over being exact at this point. A serving generally fits into a medium size hand.

Many people get very confused when it comes to understanding food labels that state protein content in terms of grams. On a scale, an ounce of meat is equal to 28 grams—but that's in *weight*. That *weight* includes the gristle, the fat, and the water. It is *not* equivalent to 28 grams of protein. (If you weigh 150 pounds, that's not equivalent to 150 pounds of muscle, nor to 150 pounds of bone, nor to 150 pounds of fat. All three are *components* of the total weight.) The conversion of *ounces* of a protein food like meat or chicken bought at the butcher's to *grams* of protein (such as you'll see on a food label) is best thought of with a mental rule I call the "rule of seven": 7 grams of protein to 1 ounce of weighed meat (or fish or poultry). That's a rough estimate, but it'll work for our purposes. So if you bought a 4-ounce steak, you're getting roughly 28 grams of protein. The reverse holds true as well. If you're using a protein shake and the label says *20 grams of protein per serving*, that's roughly equivalent to 3 ounces of a protein food like meat (20 divided by 7 is approximately 3).

Week Three: Exercise

- You're going to continue your walking program for five days a week, but you're going to increase it to 20 minutes per day.
- On the two days that you are now doing the crunches (remember, we're calling those days your "weight training" days), add the following exercise:

SQUATS (*LEGS AND BUTT*)

Stand with your arms at your sides.

Keep your feet shoulder-width apart and your head up. There can be a slight arch in your lower back (Figure 11.1).

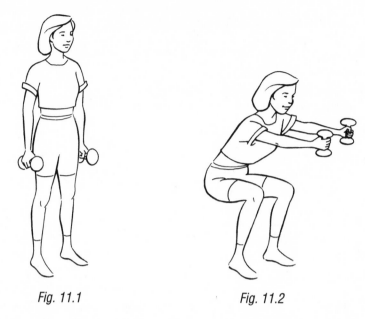

Fig. 11.1   Fig. 11.2

Slowly bend your knees while pushing your rear out, until your thighs are about parallel to the ground. Squeeze your thighs and glutes for added contraction. At the same time as you bend, bring your arms up straight in front of you for balance till they're extended straight out at shoulder height, palms facing each other (Figure 11.2).

Now come up until you're standing again, dropping your arms back to your sides as you come up, and repeat for 10–15 reps.

Don't lock your knees when you return to standing position. Adjust your foot stance until it feels comfortable.

You're going to perform one set, from 8 to 15 repetitions. (Remember that if you can do only a few repetitions to start, that's fine too—that will be your personal starting point. You'll work up to where you can do 8–15.)

To review: this is what your exercise program now looks like:

Day One	Day Two*	Day Three	Day Four*	Day Five
walk 20 min.	walk 20 min. crunches squats	walk 20 min.	walk 20 min. crunches squats	walk 20 min.

Don't forget to write down what you do in your journal.

Week Three: Self-Assessment Questionnaire

1. How much thought do you give on a day-to-day basis to your health and well-being?
2. How do you foresee your health and well-being ten years from now?
3. How much time do you normally take for yourself to take care of you?

What are the best exercises to reduce fat on my thighs and stomach?

Exercises for a specific area of the body are unfortunately pretty ineffective for reducing fat in that area. Despite what late night commercials may claim, the only fat that things like Thighmasters separate you from is any excess fat in your wallet. "Spot reducing"—the idea that you can get rid of fat by working the specific area of the body in which fat accumulates—just doesn't work. Fat won't come off the belly by doing crunches, no matter how many of them you do.

Does that mean you shouldn't do crunches? Or thigh exercises? Hardly. Besides supporting your center and helping with your posture, a good ab routine will help ensure that you'll have some muscle down there to see once the fat begins to melt away. Ditto with the thighs. But to get that fat to disappear, you'll have to do a whole lot more.

See, when you store excess fat on your body, the pattern in which it goes on is pretty much preordained by the manufacturer. As you've probably noticed, it usually seems to come off in the reverse order from which it came on (hence the old expression regarding fat: "first on, last off"). Thigh exercises will firm the muscles under the jiggle, as will ab exercises, but they won't get the jiggle off. They will however, make sure you've got some muscle tone to show when that jiggle gets reduced, and they may even help reduce some of the jiggle by making sure that untoned, loose muscles aren't contributing to the problem.

Here's what you can do to help remove the fat itself: Work all your muscles with weights, which will keep your metabolic rate up and make you a more efficient fat-burning machine. Change your diet to one built around lean protein and vegetables—no sugar, flour, or refined products. Eat a minimum of starch (and get it from oatmeal, sweet potatoes, beans and legumes) and eat only low-sugar, high-fiber fruit.

Eat double the amount of fiber you think you're eating (beans, fruits and vegetables and possibly an unsweetened fiber supplement like psyllium husks), be religious about eight to ten large glasses of pure water daily, and, as often as practical considerations permit, don't eat after 8 P.M. Add rest, relaxation, good thoughts, stress reduction, sunshine, deep breathing and a healthy dose of patience. You'll be happy with the results.

Week Four

Week Four: Journal

Continue to record feelings, thoughts, impressions, mood, food, and exercise in your journal. Just stay in communication with it. Notice what your mind puts you through over this one. Maybe you don't feel like writing— what do you think about this thought? Does it take you on a journey toward thoughts like "Maybe this whole thing is useless," "I'll never be able to do it" "the assignments are stupid"? Does it take you on a different journey? Does it take you *out* of the journey? Remember, wherever you're going with this, you're living in your head if you're engaging in this chatter. Just stay in communication with the journal.

Week Four: To-Do List

Complete at least two more tasks on the list.

Week Four: Developing Your Food Plan

- Eliminate one more food from the "B" list.
- Add one more food from the "A" list (more if you want to).

Week Four: Exercise

You're going to continue with your walking program five days a week, with the following modifications:

- Three days a week, increase to 30 minutes.
- On the two weight training days, continue walking for 20 minutes and add the following two exercises:

CHEST PRESS *(CHEST)*

Lie down on a bench, your feet resting comfortably on the floor. (If you don't have a bench you can use a step or even the floor.)

Extend your arms overhead, shoulder-width apart, palms facing out, so that the dumbbells are positioned directly over your shoulders (Figure 11.3).

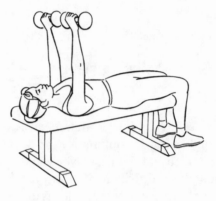

Fig. 11.3

Bend your elbows about 90 degrees, gradually lowering the weights until they are above and a little beyond your shoulders (Figure 11.4).

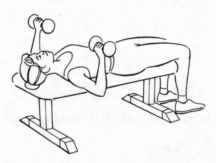

Fig. 11.4

Now push the dumbbells up with an arcing motion until they're back in starting position.

ONE-ARM ROW *(BACK)*

Bend over and rest your left hand on a bench or stool about 2.5-feet high. Extend your right leg behind you so that you're far enough away from the bench that your back is flat; make sure you don't round your back and instead keep it as flat as possible (you may actually have to arch it a little to keep it in this position). The right arm will be hanging down, straight. Your back should be like a table top in this position (Figure 11.5).

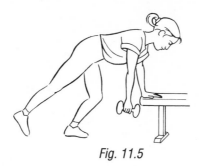

Fig. 11.5

Take a dumbell (or water bottle) in your right hand and bring it straight up toward your hip by bending your elbow and bringing it up behind you toward the ceiling (Figure 11.6). It should be almost like starting a lawn-mower in slow motion. When the weight is about at hip level, lower it back down till the arm is hanging straight down. That's one "rep." After you complete the number of reps with your right arm, reverse everything and do the same number of reps with the left arm.

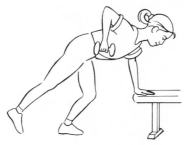

Fig. 11.6

OR

If you have access to a gym, do the "seated row" exercise (below) instead.

SEATED ROW *(BACK)*

This is done on a cable rowing machine at a gym.

Sit on the floor, feet extended, and grab the lever with both hands (Figure 11.7).

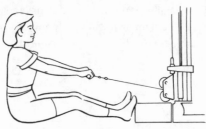

Fig. 11.7

Keep your lower back erect and bring hands and arms from an extended position back into the body.

At the completion of the movement, your hands should be just below the chest and elbows, just off the ribs (Figure 11.8).

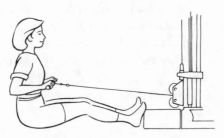

Fig. 11.8

You're going to perform one set of each of these exercises (the chest press and either the one-arm row or the seated row), consisting of anywhere from 8 to 15 repetitions. (Remember that if you can only do a few repetitions in the beginning, that's fine too—that will be your personal starting point. You'll work up to where you can do 8–15.)

To review: Your weight training days (twice a week, after walking) will now consist of four exercises: crunches (10–20 reps), the squat, the chest press and the row (one set each, 8–15 repetitions per set). Rest only as much as you need to between exercises.

Here's what the week will now look like:

Day One	Day Two	Day Three	Day Four	Day Five
walk 30 min.	walk 20 min. crunches squats chest press row	walk 30 min.	walk 20 min. crunches squats chest press row	walk 30 min.

Don't forget to take a few minutes after every workout and relax. Stretch, decompress, chill out. And make sure you tell your journal what you did.

Week Four: Self-Assessment Questionnaire

1. What, if anything, would you most like to change about your life?
2. How could you accomplish this?

By the way, I just want to remind you that there's no "right" way to do these exercises or answer these questions. So if, for example, the only way you can imagine changing some aspect of your life means being whimsical or doing something outrageous, go ahead and write it down. Maybe it'll be something concrete you could do, maybe it'll be something completely fanciful. Who cares? Make it up. And don't judge what you put on the paper.

And speaking of judging, it's time to talk a bit about those little voices we all have living inside our heads.

Using the Scale to Set Goals

The scale is a tool. And like any tool it can be employed in an empowering way or in a destructive way. If you use the scale as a general reality check and don't give it too much power over your life, if you don't allow it to become a measure of your success or personal worth, if you don't use it as something to become obsessed with and beat yourself up with, then the scale is a fine tool to help you check in and see how you're doing in a general way. If you set goals as a game and have fun with them, great. If you set goals and then consistently cause yourself anxiety about whether or not you're achieving them fast enough, then you're headed for trouble.

People lose weight at different rates. They grow up at different rates, they develop skills at different rates, they learn life's lessons at different rates. If you honor this, and never let it be far from your mind, you will naturally set goals that are empowering for you.

Goals—and the scale—are great. Just make sure *you* are in charge of them. *You* run the goals; they don't run you.

SCIENCE, SEX, AND THE HIGH-PROTEIN DIET

Stupid Media Tricks: "She Blinded Me With Science"

The truth is more important than the facts.

—FRANK LLOYD WRIGHT

In our own not-so-distant past, people didn't have to struggle with such messy issues as right and wrong or good and evil. They had the church to do it for them. If the church said something was bad you didn't do it, and if it said it was OK then no problem. We willingly surrendered our powers to judge things for ourselves, preferring the security of trusting it to the experts who had a direct line to God. In many parts of the world it remains that way today. Whether church, shaman, ayatollah or rabbi, the word is handed down and people blindly obey. It's certainly easier that way. No muss, no fuss, no messy evaluations, no angst, no worry, no insecurity.

In the modern world, we too have abdicated our powers to decide, evaluate and think critically about anything we don't understand fully, except now we listen to the authorities of a different church: The Church of Science. I call this Scientism.

There are two dangers with science: believing that it can prove *nothing* and believing that it can prove *everything*.

You need to know this, and know it well, because the word "science" is being used to sell you anything and everything from food to dietary concepts, and much of it—the products *and* the ideas—is junk. We buy into all this because we suffer from a mass delusion—a blind, almost religious faith among ordinary people in both of the following two concepts: One,

145

there are such things as neutral, scientific facts, and two, everyone agrees on their meaning.

Suppose a handyman came to your house to do some repair work, and he brought with him his favorite soldering iron. Now that's fine if you need some electrical work done, but suppose your wooden chair needs a new leg. That soldering iron can be the best soldering iron in the world, but it's the wrong tool for the job. Our experts have become so enamored of their methods that they have convinced us that if we can't measure something or demonstrate it by their favorite designs, it must not exist. And the research methods our scientists have come to love and rely on are not always the perfect—or only—way to get good information.

The research method they've come to love the most—considered the gold standard for scientific investigation—is something called the "double-blind, randomized, crossover study." Without going into too much statistical gobbledygook, let me give you a simple example of what that looks like. You want to test the effects of a new weight loss drug on appetite. So you get some rats who have been genetically bred to be virtually identical, and you randomly split them into two groups. You give both groups free access to the same rat food. Before starting the experiment you measure how much they eat normally. Then you give one group of rats the appetite-suppressing drug, and the other group something called a placebo, which is basically an inert substance that doesn't do anything. You do this because it's been found that the very act of giving a treatment, drug, injection, pill or food has effects of its own (especially in people), so you want to make sure any difference in appetite you may observe between the two groups is purely because of the drug. You don't tell the volunteer college students who feed the rats their respective pills whether they are feeding them the weight loss drug or the placebo, because it has also been found (especially with people) that the experimenter's expectations can have a huge effect on the outcome. This way no one knows anything. Then, at the end of the experiment, you again measure how much the two groups of rats are eating and examine the data to see if in fact there are any meaningful differences in the amount of food the two groups ate. If the group getting the weight loss drug really eats a lot less, you've got yourself a publishable study.

Oh were it only that simple.

This model—a single event (drug) being measured against a single outcome (rat food consumption)—works very well indeed for the investigation of some things, but is quite unsuited for many others. Nutrients, for example, do not work as isolated compounds—they work synergistically, and testing a single nutrient on a person who has a complex and sometimes baffling array of symptoms is not necessarily going to reveal what that nutrient is capable of doing when it's properly and artfully combined with others in a program that's specifically tailored to that individual's needs. A pesticide or toxin tested in a "one drug/ one effect" study may be found "safe" by the FDA, but that hardly begins to tell us about the effect of a much more typical exposure to a massive amount of different toxins in unpredictable and bewildering combinations, particularly in the system of an individual who might have some deficiencies in certain detoxifying enzymes. We shouldn't assume, therefore, as mainstream medicine often does, that because there aren't yet convincing studies of an effect that the effect doesn't exist.

Yet that's exactly what the medical establishment does all the time when they ignore clinical experience and observation and stubbornly say, Jerry McGuire–like, "Show me the studies." Anyone who has ever eaten a food only to feel bloated or fatigued knows darn well that *something* is going on, even if the tests show he's not technically allergic. Anyone who has ever found herself utterly unable to lose weight and tired all the time knows darn well that *something* is going on, even if her thyroid tests come back normal. And anyone who has ever suffered through a myriad of unbearable mood swings during her period knows that *something* is not right even if her tests don't show anything. But scientists think that if you can't measure it, it's not worth talking about, or worse, it doesn't exist. That's why they have solemn conferences in which they assure themselves that there's no such thing as Gulf War syndrome or multiple chemical sensitivities; that's why women have been told by their doctors for eons that PMS is "all in their heads"; that's why until recently you could hardly find an orthodox M.D. who thought there was such a thing as fibromyalgia; and that's why, as a rule, scientists are sure that animals don't have feelings.

But don't get me started.

Imagine, if you will, a courtroom. You have a case to present that involves an elephant. The judge says, "I don't believe you, Mr. Jones. There *is* no elephant."

You reply, "Well, as a matter of fact, Your Honor, there is. Not only that, but if it please the court, I have him right outside." (In fact, right on the courtroom steps, attracting quite an admiring crowd, is the elephant in question.)

"Well, bring him in," says the judge. "I'm willing to be convinced. I'm open-minded. I'll take a look at him."

"Sorry, Your Honor," you say, "he won't fit through the door. But if you'll just come outside the building here to take a peek, you can see him for yourself. He's right outside."

"No, young man," says the judge. "Any evidence must be brought before me in this courtroom. Those are the rules of evidence."

"But Your Honor," you protest, "*he won't fit through the door.*"

"Then he must not exist," says the judge. "Until I can see him myself *in my courtroom*, I must rule that there is no such thing as an elephant."

Believe it or not, this *Alice in Wonderland* situation is just what many of us who recommend nutritional supplements, lower carbohydrate intake, herbal medicine or natural foods diets are dealing with every day. It's not that the recommendations don't work. It's that they cannot always be demonstrated with the narrow, one-dimensional technique that "science"—Western science—insists on as "proof." We have a big gray elephant sitting outside the courtroom that won't fit through the door. We need to stop dismissing his existence and start thinking about how to design a bigger courtroom door.

The use of scientific tools and measurements is a great addition to the repertory of observation and deduction, and it allows us to see and measure things in ways we couldn't otherwise do. But these tools were always meant to be an *addition* to the repertory—they were never meant as a replacement for old-fashioned intuition, experience, wisdom, judgment, and common sense. Yet we have turned all those wonderful innate powers over to experts to such a degree that we no longer trust our own abilities to simply observe the world. We've replaced the church with our new god—the god of science. As Carol Simontacchi, author of *The Crazy Makers*, says, "Our obsessive need to check with the experts before we sit down to a meal is unique to this century." Maybe it's time to take another look at the wholesale surrender of our own powers of judgment and observation and to examine a little more closely this new church of ours, "Science," and our blind faith in it.

Why, in television commercials for a car battery, does the pitchman talking to you in front of the auto-parts store wear a lab coat? Is he wearing the lab coat so the blood from the brain surgery he's doing back there won't splatter on his suit? No, he's wearing it because the people who make the product—any product, in fact—want to capitalize on the fact that the American public has a propensity to buy absolutely any information that is delivered by someone in a white lab coat and a serious expression who begins a sentence by deeply intoning, "Studies show . . ." Look, I hate to break this to you, but not everyone doing "studies" is a Jonas Salk or an Albert Einstein laboring tirelessly for the good of humanity. And not all studies are not created equal. I promise you that I could create a well-designed study that would stand up to rigorous scientific scrutiny from which you could conclude that M&Ms were a weight loss food. All I'd have to do is take some very overweight people, put them on a rigorously controlled program of exercise and a low-calorie regimen of vegetables, fruit, grilled fish and a daily handful of M&Ms, and if they lost weight—which they probably would—I could absolutely say that "M&Ms, *when used as part of a healthy program of diet and exercise,* helped people to lose a significant amount of weight." Think you don't hear that kind of thing on television on a daily basis?

To understand better how to think a little more critically the next time you hear a pronouncement about what "scientific studies show," I need you to understand something called the "confounding variable."

Ever see a really good staged professional wrestling match? At the height of the frenzy, with the crowd screaming, the "villain" will often reach into his trunks for some secret weapon, like a blackjack, out of "sight" of the referee, and then smash it into his opponent's face. The crowd screams and points to the trunks signaling the referee to look, but the referee runs around and can't "see" anything so he doesn't "disqualify" the villain. The villain does it again, to the screams of the crowd, and then quickly sticks the weapon back into his trunks. He makes a hands-up gesture and a face of mock innocence to the referee while the fans are screaming "Look in his trunks, look in his trunks!" Eventually the villain wins the match.

The blackjack is a "confounding variable."

In any experimental design, there is always the possibility of some unseen or unaccounted-for variable influencing the results. We're going to see this later when we talk about some of the epidemiological studies of protein and disease, but for now I'm going to give you a great example that actually happened to me in graduate school. Some psychologists, worried that they weren't getting enough male student volunteers for experiments, wanted to see whether more students would sign up if they offered them a choice of two locations, uptown or downtown. They thought that maybe the downtown location of the sign-up office was too inconvenient. So they added an uptown location—Professor Smith's office—as an additional sign-up site. Sure enough, the number of male volunteers started noticeably increasing at the uptown sign-up location. In fact, at a rather amazing rate. There was no increase in the rate of sign-up at the downtown location, but virtually every available time slot for volunteering was filled at the uptown location. The conclusion? Must be that offering that uptown location really made a difference. Must be that the downtown location was more of an inconvenience than anyone had previously suspected. Sounds reasonable, doesn't it?

Until some graduate students decided to do a little further investigation. They went up to the uptown office of Professor Smith. It turns out that his secretary was a virtual look-alike of Pamela Anderson. They found her surrounded by what seemed like half the male class, joking, flirting, showing off, talking and signing up in droves for whatever she was offering.

The gorgeous secretary was the confounding variable. Unexpected, unaccounted for, and strongly, powerfully influencing the results of what looked like a perfectly objective study.

Even in academia, and even with the loftiest of intentions and intellectual rigor, some studies are highly flawed because *the assumptions on which they are based are not accurate.* Let me give you some examples of why a study might draw the wrong conclusion because the assumptions it was based on were incorrect.

Suppose a researcher wants to see if our old friends, the fatty acids EPA and DHA, are effective in treating depression. You may recall from Chapter 10 that these fatty acids are made by the body from the raw material of *another* fatty acid, alpha-linolenic acid (ALA). The body takes ALA, which consists of an eighteen carbon chain containing three double bonds, and goes to work on it. Enzymes elongate it by adding more carbons to the chain, and other enzymes desaturate it by adding more chemical glue called "double bonds." Eventually, in the best of all possible worlds, it is transformed into those superstar fatty acids, the twenty and twenty-two carbon chains called, respectively, EPA and DHA. Now it's long been assumed that if you get enough of that raw material, alpha-linolenic acid, you will be assured of getting your EPA and DHA. So when our researcher gives his subjects ALA, he assumes he will actually be measuring the effects of more EPA and DHA on depressive symptoms. But that assumption may be wrong. The numerous chemical reactions that need to take place to convert ALA into DHA and EPA do not happen efficiently, effectively, or sometimes *at all* with many people. If our researcher gave the subjects in his study ALA (assuming it converts perfectly well to the fatty acids in question), he might very well draw the conclusion that these wonderful fatty acids (DHA and EPA) do nothing for depression. What in fact might have happened is that the raw materials never got transformed into DHA and EPA in the first place.

Here's another example of how omitting a crucial consideration can produce worthless results. Suppose I want to do a study to find out if listening to music while on a treadmill makes people run faster or longer or enjoy their workouts more. Unfortunately, though, I don't know much about music nor about the taste of my subjects. So I go out and get some

Beethoven; I put one group of subjects on the treadmill and let them listen to the String Quartet op. 101 while they run; the other group runs in silence. And guess what? There is *no difference* in speed, distance or enjoyment. My conclusion: *Listening to music makes no difference in running performance on the treadmill.*

But wait, you say. There's a problem with that study. You only gave them one kind of music; that's not a fair test. Point taken, say I. So in the interest of fairness, I go out and get a musical smorgasbord: classical, opera, country and fifties rock and roll. I redo the study, and guess what? *Still absolutely no difference.* In fact, the music-listening runners actually enjoyed their workouts *less* and got off the treadmill *faster* than the control group who didn't listen at all.

On the surface of it this may look like a very rigorous, well-designed study, but let's take a closer look. My subjects were twenty-year-old college students. Although the four categories of music may have been different from one another to *my* ears, in all likelihood they fell into the *same* category for my *subjects*, and this category was "*I hate this stuff!*" Had I been more astute in my study design, I might have offered hip-hop, or rap, or metal as a category, which is far more likely to speak to my population of twenty-year-old subjects, and I might have gotten entirely different results and drawn a completely different conclusion about the power of music to affect exercise.

This happens *all the time* in peer-reviewed, published studies. If the wrong form of a supplement is used, for example, or it's not used in conjunction with the right supporting nutrients, or it's used on the wrong population, the study result may well show no effect of the supplement. (And you can be sure the "anti-vitamin" brigade will trot that study out at every opportunity.) For instance, a recent study in England concluded that chromium supplementation had no effect on glucose tolerance in patients with type ll diabetes; yet, when I looked at the study, I saw that the researchers had used a dosage of 100 mcg of chromium, a paltry amount that no one familiar with the action of chromium would *expect* to have an effect (most studies use between 200 and 1,000 mcg, with the best results usually gained from the higher amounts).

The situation is made even more troublesome when politics gets into the picture and big money is at stake. With thousands of studies published, it's relatively easy (and all too common) to selectively pay attention to the studies that support your position and ignore the ones that don't. Research is much like the Bible—it can be interpreted in a lot of different ways and can be invoked to support a myriad of different positions. More often than you might imagine, scientists—who, after all, are also human—make their minds up about something first and then selectively look for the studies that support that position.

So just as you don't rush out and buy stock in every single company that announces it's going public, you shouldn't buy into every concept that's marketed to you because it has "studies" to support it. Furthermore, you're rarely getting the study results from the horse's mouth—you're getting it from a reporter who barely understood it in the first place and tried to condense it into a sound byte that would get your attention. Trust me on this.

Now, am I bashing science? Absolutely not. I have the greatest respect for scientific investigation when it's used wisely, in the quest for wisdom (though I am much less in awe of *statistics*). I am, however, bashing dumbness and marketing and ossified thinking, especially when they're used in the service of making you less healthy than you could be.

What about "the facts" of nutrition and healthy diets about which there seems to be such profound disagreement? Well, I've got more bad news. Nutrition facts are pretty neutral pieces of information. There are absolutely zillions of them, and by themselves, they're not of much value. They can be arranged in almost any order to support a limitless number of hypotheses, theories and conclusions. Like crayons in a box, the picture they produce is only as good as the artist using them. *Facts are only as useful as the conclusions we allow ourselves to draw from them.* The facts *don't* "speak for themselves," or at least not very well. They need a voice with wisdom and vision to assemble them in the right way so they can reveal their message.

We're going to come back to this in Chapter 20, when I talk about some personal facts in *your* life and the emotional meaning and power that that *you've* given them. But for now, let's concentrate on scientific, objective "facts" and how they can be manipulated, even by well-meaning people, to support a conclusion that's not always justified. Such as, for example, the conclusion that "the high carbohydrate food pyramid is a good way for you to eat," or "calories are all that count," or "you will get cancer and heart disease if you add more high quality protein and fat to your diet."

So the next time you hear a celebrity with a great body interviewed about her diet, or the next time some "expert" tells you that vegetarian diets protect against disease, the question you should always be asking yourself is this: *What else might be going on here?*

A few years ago, one of the great heavyweight boxers was Evander Holyfield. Holyfield might just have been one of the most perfect specimens of muscle and sinew and conditioning and athletic performance seen in the later half of the twentieth century. Now it just so happened that I spoke with a reliable source in Holyfield's training camp and you know what Holyfield's absolute favorite food was?

You ready?

French fries.

Fact one: Holyfield is in great shape. Fact two: He eats french fries. So what's the take-home point from that? If you want to have a great body like Holyfield you should eat french fries? Now that may sound ridiculous, but believe me, that is *exactly* the reasoning that marketers use when they sell you products, and that, unfortunately, many scientists use when they draw conclusions from unexamined "facts" about how people eat.

Facts don't tell you everything. Whether in detective work, science or nutrition it's the *connections* between the facts that count. It's the conclusions that facts allow you to draw that make them valuable. Facts are neutral observations and are only as useful as the conclusions they allow us to draw from them, and that's where the "art" in "art and science" comes in.

And it's entirely possible for good people to agree completely on the facts while coming to completely different conclusions about what they mean. Here's one of my favorite examples, a story told by Drs. Michael and Mary Dan Eades, who have been fighting the good fight against the nutritional establishment for over a dozen years: A young boy goes running to his father. "Daddy, Daddy," he cries, "come quick! The stable boy is in the barn with Sis, and they're taking their pants down! Come quick, Daddy," he urges, "*they're going to pee all over the hay!*" As the father gets his shotgun, he calmly says to the boy, "Son, you got your facts straight. But I disagree with your conclusion!"

Epidemiological studies of nutrition—which are basically huge observational studies that look at a zillion things like diet, median age, climate, population, race, exercise patterns of the citizenry, voting behavior—*describe* things. They observe what happens, they state facts and describe associations, but the *conclusions* that they draw from these facts—the theories they put forth about why things are associated with each other—are often far from perfect. For example, many studies have concluded that high protein intake is to blame for the high incidence of cancer and heart disease associated with the standard American diet. But a closer look at this association reveals that perhaps this common conclusion is no more accurate than the conclusion of the little boy who thought his sis was going to pee in the hay. Why? Well, let's take a closer look at the characteristics of the standard American diet that is so clearly associated with a greater risk for cancer and heart disease and diabetes.

Recently I found myself in Las Vegas, at one of the all-you-can-eat buffets. Go some time, it's an education. Or go to Disneyland. Or any cruise ship. Look around at what people pile on their plates. Look at the *quality* of food, and then at the *quantity* of food. It is unprecedented in human history. Mounds and mounds of dripping, saucy, sweetened, creamy, pulverized, overcooked, processed "food products," in portions that would feed a small starving family in Ethiopia for a week. *That* is the standard American diet. Of *course* it is linked with virtually every degenerative disease commonly seen in Western societies. But do not, please, blame that association on protein. Don't fall into the trap of believing that because there is a lot of protein in that junk food orgy that passes for a diet that every horrible thing that is *associated* with the diet is due to the *protein* in it. Here are a few *other* things that are true about the standard American diet and, in fact, the diets of most Westernized, industrial countries on the planet:

- Most of the protein in it is from factory-farmed animals that are loaded with antibiotics, hormones and steroids and force-fed a grain-based diet entirely different from what these animals would graze on or eat in the wild.
- A huge amount of the protein in the diet comes from processed meats such as cold cuts and hot dogs, which are filled with carcinogens like nitrates.
- These large amounts of processed, toxic protein sources are coupled with very low amounts of vegetables.
- Ditto for fruit.
- Ditto for fiber.
- The diet also contains an extremely *high* intake of trans-fatty acids, a particularly insidious kind of man-made, mutated fat that is beginning to be identified as probably the most dangerous of the dietary fats.
- The diet also contains an extremely *low* amount of the valuable long chain fatty acids such as DHA in comparison to the high intake of saturated fats and refined vegetable oils.
- The diet contains an extremely *high* amount of sugar.
- The diet is a virtual recipe for high and unbalanced levels of insulin production.

That, my friends, in a nutshell is the standard American diet that you and I have been eating, and it is the diet that is associated with higher risks for virtually every disease and condition that you don't want to have. My question for you is this:

Is it *protein* in the diet that is causing the mischief? Because that is what the diet "dictocrats" would like you to believe, and it is unequivocally wrong-headed. What you have here is a combination of factors that are a prescription for bad health. *There is absolutely no reason to think that a diet built around high-quality protein plus a ton of vegetables and a healthy amount of traditional, nourishing fats would do anything other than have a positive effect on health.* I am waiting for a study, any study, that shows that consuming high-quality, non-toxic protein balanced with phytonutrient and fiber-rich vegetables, a moderate amount of low-sugar fruit like berries and a reasonable amount of heart healthy fats from nuts, avocados, fish and olives is associated with a higher risk of disease. It'll be a long wait. In the meantime, please put this in with those tattoos under your eyelids:

There are no such studies. They don't exist. All the studies that have shown a deleterious effect of high-protein diets have compared diets high in junk protein and low in vegetables and fruits (the standard American diet) to diets high in vegetables and fruits and low in protein and good fats. The Shape Up program is built on protein, good fat, a ton of vegetables and some fruit; the only things it's low in are starch, sugar, and junk.

It's important that you understand this, because in the Shape Up program, I *am* telling you to eat more protein (and probably more fat) than you're used to eating. I'm also recommending that you eat fewer carbohydrates than you're probably used to eating. This does not make Shape Up a high-protein diet, and it certainly doesn't make it dangerous. But here's what I promise you: Some journalist will get hold of some doctor with an agenda who doesn't know what he's talking about, and that doctor will go on the news and talk about all the dangers of high-protein diets, and inevitably the Shape Up program will be lumped in with them.

Forewarned is forearmed, so let's take some time and define our terms.

Sex and the High-Protein Diet

Sir, I have found you an argument,
but I am not obliged to find you an understanding.

—*DR. JOHNSON*

There's a great scene in the classic Woody Allen movie *Annie Hall*. In the movie, Alvie Singer (played by Woody) and his girlfriend Annie (played by Dianne Keaton) are both in therapy with different therapists. In the scene I'm talking about there's a split screen, and you see both characters with their respective shrinks. On the left side, Alvie is saying to his shrink, "We hardly ever have sex!" The therapist asks, "Well, how often do you have sex?" and Alvie moans, "Only three times a week." Over on the right side of the screen you see Annie complaining to her shrink, "He wants to have sex all the time!" Her therapist asks, "Well, how often do you have sex?" and Annie wails, "All the time! Three times a week!"

Which brings us to low-carb diets. And to the question of definitions.

I'm frequently asked about high-protein/low-carbohydrate diets, and the thing I'm always struck by is that when I ask the person posing the question how he defines "high-protein" the answer sounds a lot like the scene from *Annie Hall*. What constitutes "low" or "high" protein (or low- or high-carbohydrate) really depends on what your reference point is. Time and time again I hear speakers and writers who should know better misrepresent such dietary plans as The Zone, characterizing it as a "high-protein" diet. Why is it misrepresentation? Because Dr. Barry Sears (author of *The Zone*) and other advocates of this strategy, such as Ann Louise Gittleman, recommend a dietary distribution of 40 percent carbohydrates, 30 percent protein and 30 percent fat. If you notice, the lion's share of calories in this plan comes from carbohydrates (40 percent)! Is that a high-protein diet? Well, if you're a government agency or a traditionally trained dietitian and you believe that folks should consume only 12 percent of their calories from protein, sure it is. I guess how you look at it depends on what side of the split screen you're sitting on.

The dietary guidelines I recommend in the Shape Up program do not really constitute a low-carb diet, although the American Dietary Association zealots might disagree. To them, a recommendation that carbohydrates constitute anything less than 55–65 percent of your daily calories is defined as "low." Personally, I think they're nuts.

The high-carbohydrate diet recommended by most of the powers that be in the nutrition establishment and represented by the USDA food pyramid *doesn't work* for most people, and certainly doesn't work for weight loss. Never has, never will. It's the biggest uncontrolled experiment in nutritional history, and it's led to, among other things, a pandemic of type II diabetes—once a relatively rare disease seen only in late adulthood, now cropping up with scary regularity among fifteen-year-olds—and has contributed to a host of other degenerative diseases. Have some people lost weight on it? Sure. And if you happen to be in the quartile of the population who is gifted with the ability to metabolize carbohydrates optimally, who normally secrete insulin or who is genetically suited to this kind of eating (the Bantu of South Africa, for example) and simply got fat by eating too much food, you may be able to correct that and do OK on a high-carb regimen. But I doubt it. The chances of you being in that group, statistically, are small. And if you're reading this book, I'd say the chances are virtually zero.

Why is it terribly unlikely that a high-carbohydrate diet will work for you? Because unless you're one of the lucky ones in the population whose metabolism operates flawlessly, who is not struggling with a weight problem, who is eating whole and unrefined foods, who is getting adequate intake of fiber, who has no discernible food intolerances or hypersensitivies, who is exercising daily, has little insulin insensitivity, seems to process a high-grain-based diet effortlessly and has no serious disturbances in blood sugar levels, you're gonna have a problem with the typical American high-carb/low-fat diet. In a word, it's going to make you fat. Why? Because in the rage to hang horns on the villain and banish fat from the American diet, we have wound up replacing it with something just as bad—far more carbohydrates than our Paleolithic digestive systems were ever designed to process. Furthermore, those carbs are not the "good" kind that well-meaning nutritionists talk about when they urge us to eat more of them. They're processed, refined, full of hidden sugars, loaded with potential allergens, made with bleached and processed flours, devoid of nutrients and loaded with calories. These foods may be low in fat, but they're making us sick and they're making us fat.

The dietary guidelines in the Shape Up program were designed for weight loss, but more important, they were also designed for health. Sure, there are people who will be able to eat more starches or fruit than are on the recommended lists (and there will be many who will have to eat less), but that's what individualizing and customizing a strategy is all about. Sure, the percentage of calories coming from carbohydrates is a bit less than politically correct zealots would have you believe you should be eating, but if the official, government-approved version of what you should be eating was working so well for you, you probably wouldn't be reading this book in the first place.

So, you ask, does that make the Shape Up plan another of those high-protein diets I've been reading so much about, that are supposed to be so dangerous?

Well, before I answer you, I'd like to tell you one of my favorite stories. I call it "Jonny's Movie Parable."

Four friends run into each other outside the movie sixplex in the mall, just as the show is letting out. "Wow, some movie," says the first. "Did you like it?" The second says, "I thought that was one of the saddest things I've ever seen." The third says, "Sad? Are you kidding? I thought it was a riot! Didn't you get the humor in it?" The fourth says, "You guys, you're completely missing the point! The whole thing was about the cinematic technique, and the whole point wasn't whether it was funny or sad, it was the use of the visuals!" This conversation continues on for quite a while, with points being made on each side, the argument getting increasingly heated and belligerent until they suddenly realize . . .

They all saw different movies.

I always remember the movie parable whenever I'm about to launch into a discussion about a controversial subject like high-protein diets, because I have frequently found that though everyone in the discussion *assumes* we're talking about the same thing, in fact everyone has a very different idea of what constitutes the subject on the table. The first order of business has always got to be this: *make sure everybody's talking about the same movie!*

So let's talk a little about this so-called "high-protein" diet. And by the way, if you'd like to skip the rest of this section, here's the punch line: The Shape Up program, *by any reasonable definition you can come up with,* is *not* a "high-protein" diet. It *is* a protein-rich (or protein-adequate) program. It will *not* cause kidney disease, it will *not* deplete your bones of important minerals, and it will *not* cause you to go into the dreaded (and highly misrepresented) state of ketosis and curl up in a bundle and die.

Now if you want to know more about where we *got* all these misconceptions about high-protein diets in the first place, read on.

Pretend for a moment that a bunch of professional sexologists got together in the towers of academia, or wherever it is that professional sexologists get together, and decided to write a position paper on modern sexual behavior.

They looked at all kinds of people—nuns, teenagers, old people in rest homes, single people, married people, gays, straights, rabbis, priests, sexual athletes and sexual phobics, the religious right, Libertarians, Republicans, Democrats, fishermen, accountants, virtually anyone living in America at the beginning of the twenty-first century.

Heavily influenced by the mores and community standards of the time, by the prevailing sensibilities, by the raw data in their statistics, and trying as best as they could to come up with a joint statement that took into account every possible situation and circumstance, that represented the statistical average and satisfied as many of the panel participants as possible, they declared the following compromise:

"Normal sexual behavior means having heterosexual sex once every two weeks with your partner to whom you are married."

By the same token, here are the corollaries of this statement: Anything *less* than this standard is "low-sex behavior"; anything *more* than this is "high sex behavior."

Sound ridiculous?

Welcome to the world of the nutrition establishment.

Because, ladies and gentleman of the jury, to the diet dictocrats a "high-protein diet" means nothing more than a diet in which you eat more protein than the American Dietetic Association and the United States Department of Agriculture *think* you should be eating. And we can't even begin to talk about whether that "high" protein diet is healthy or not until we ask the question "Was the original recommendation a good one, and *for whom?*"

So we have all these folks going around talking about "high-protein" diets and their dangers, misrepresenting eating programs that are completely safe and completely healthy as being "high-protein," simply because these programs recommend more protein than the powers that be think a normal, average person should be eating.

And no one has bothered to ask, "Could the powers that be have been wrong in the first place?"

To which I would reply, They are about as right as the prescription that everyone should have sex once every two weeks with their married partner.

Does this mean having sex once every two weeks with your married partner is "wrong"? Heck no. In fact, it might be *exactly right*—for *some people.* But it *does* mean that if you think this is a hard and fast rule for the "proper" way to have sex, you might have been visiting another planet for the last few decades. At the very least, you've never seen *Oprah*, let alone *Jerry Springer.*

The USDA and the American Dietetic Association think that the "right" way for you to eat is for you to take in about 12 percent of your calories from protein. Anything more is a high-protein diet. *Well it's only high if you accept the 12-percent standard as the normal or correct one, which is much like accepting the "once every two weeks" maxim as the "normal and correct" mode for sexual expression.*

Please remember this the next time the subject of "high-protein" diets comes up. It's only "high" if you accept 12 percent as "normal." I hope, as we move through this book, that you will begin to question the blind acceptance of this amount as "universally right" for everyone.

So the next time someone asks you if you're on a "high-protein" diet, think of that scene in *Annie Hall.*

And then ask them, "Compared to what?"

WEEKS FIVE AND SIX

Week Five

Week Five: Journal

Keep writing.

Oh, and by the way. . . once in a while, when you're sure you have no more to write about, nothing more to say. . .

. . . keep writing.

Week Five: To-Do List

Two more things come off the list.

Noticing anything? Write it down in your journal.

Week Five: Developing Your Food Plan

Now we're going to start paying a little closer attention to our carbohydrate intake. It's time to start fine-tuning. If you're not noticing any changes yet, or even if you are, it's time to adjust that carbohydrate intake from the "B" list and bring it down a little further. Nothing ridiculous, mind you. Just look at it like a budget you're trying to trim. Where's the excess? Start cutting it down.

Week Five: Exercise

Time to up the walking program. Two days a week go to 45 minutes a day. One day a week, stay at 30. The remaining two days, when you weight train, continue at 20. So a typical week will look like this:

Day One	Day Two	Day Three	Day Four	Day Five
walk 45 min.	walk 20 min. weight training	walk 30 min.	walk 20 min. weight training	walk 45 min.

On your two weight training days, add the following two exercises:

BICEP CURL (ARMS)

Stand with a pair of dumbbells in your hands, palms facing out and feet shoulder-width apart (Figure 13.1).

Keeping your elbows stable, raise the dumbbells toward your shoulders (Figure 13.2) and then bring them slowly back down (Figure 13.1). Repeat for 8 to 12 reps.

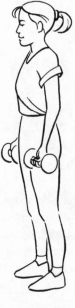

Fig. 13.1

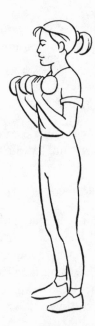

Fig. 13.2

TRICEP DIPS (ARMS)

Sit on the edge of a bench or step, with your hands on the edge of the bench and fingers facing forward (Figure. 13.3).

Lift your butt off the bench and lower it toward the floor by bending your arms at the elbows. Make sure you stay perpendicular to the ground, back straight. Don't push the hips forward (Figure 13.4).

Lift yourself back up by straightening your arms, but don't rest your butt back on the bench until you're done. Repeat for 8–12 reps.

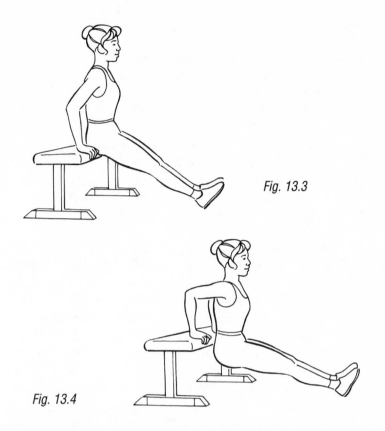

Fig. 13.3

Fig. 13.4

So to review the weight training portion of this week, you will now be doing six exercises: crunches, the squat, the chest press, the row, the bicep curl and the tricep dip. On those two weight training days I want you to do one set each of these six exercises, in sequence.

Day One	Day Two	Day Three	Day Four	Day Five
walk 30 min.	walk 20 min. crunches squats bench press row bicep curls tricep dips	walk 30 min.	walk 20 min. crunches squats bench press row bicep curls tricep dips	walk 30 min.

Then finish your workout with some relaxing stretches.

Week Five: Self-Assessment Questionnaire

This week, you're going to answer two questions:

1. What's the *one thing* you most dislike about your body?

And, more important,

2. How would your life be different if—and when—you could change that?

(By the way, if you think this is a trick question, you're partly right.) Give it a little thought before you continue with this section.

Back already? OK, I'm going to let you in on a secret formula that I think will help you shed a little light on the subject. I call it "the Bowden Equation" and it goes like this:

Expectation – Reality = Disappointment.

We're rarely made happy or sad by actual events, whether it be pounds lost, increase in income, or winning second place in the "Most Improved Body" contest. What makes us happy or sad is the *story* we make up in our heads about the event. Let's say the "event" is that you lost two pounds. If you're unhappy with that, it's because you've got a "story" made up about it that says, "I lost five pounds but I *should have lost ten*," which is a story guaranteed to produce disappointment. Take the same five pounds lost, however, with a story that goes, "Two pounds would've been great and, *wow, I lost five*" and—voilà—the resulting feeling is entirely different.

Think you'd be happy with a ten-thousand-dollar raise? Most of us would be . . . *unless* . . .

. . . you were hoping for twenty.

Does this mean you shouldn't aim high? Shouldn't go for the gold? Course not. But what it *does* mean is that you need to dream with your eyes wide open. If you've been two hundred pounds all your adult life and you decide to really get in shape and you lose twenty pounds, I think that's a victory. I think it's a triumph and I think it's an achievement, and I think you're ripping yourself off if you don't acknowledge that and allow yourself to enjoy it. But if you're thinking that it's a failure because you still don't look like Kate Moss or Brad Pitt, well . . .

You've got some serious rethinking to do, my friend.

You've been on the Shape Up Program for five weeks now. What could you find about the transformations that you've made in your body, in the way you feel, in your fitness level or even in the way you look at things that would allow you to feel good right now? What would it take for that to happen?

Write it in your journal.

To break out of a continual cycle of disappointment and frustration that many of us get trapped in, we need to take a look at not just what *isn't* happening—to our bodies, our careers, our relationships and our lives—but also at what *is* happening and what we *expect* to happen. When you stop concentrating so much on the end result, two things start to happen: One, you'll find you can enjoy the journey a lot more. And two, ironically enough, the results come much faster.

Shedding Pounds Quickly

Suppose you were in a seminar on financial prosperity, and you overheard the following conversation between two students: One student says, "I'm here because I really want to take charge of my financial life. I have goals and dreams, and I want to learn how to make them reality. I want to learn how to grow a business, make a difference, create value for my customers and create wealth for my family, and I'll do whatever it takes to get there." The second student says, "I need to make a million bucks in a week. I want them to tell me what I should do." Which student would your intuition tell you has a better chance of getting rich?

I think of that every time someone tells me they "have" to lose weight really fast. It saddens me, because I know from experience that whatever they wind up doing is not going to work, and they'll be back asking that same question a year from now. The fact is there's no fast way to lose fat, and anyone who tells you there is is lying. The only way to lose weight quickly is to either get very sick, take drugs, or starve, and I'm not interested in any of those strategies. I've also found that when a person has a lot of desperation around the issue of weight loss, there's a lot of other stuff going on as well that should be addressed. After all, most people who want to lose weight *really* want to be happier. So why not work on being happier at the same time as you work on changing your body? That way you can enjoy the process and the journey a lot more, and maybe even get some results you hadn't anticipated.

The body can only drop about two pounds of fat a week, more or less. That's not to say that people don't often lose more dramatic amounts, especially in the beginning of a new program. Part of the reason is that many of us have undetected sensitivities to foods we routinely eat, and these foods may be causing us to retain what is sometimes called "false fat," the unpleasant bloating and water retention that comes from eating foods to which you are hypersensitive. Since many diet plans remove or limit wheat, which is a prime offender in the food sensitivity arena, there is often a more rapid reduction in scale weight at first.

I urge anyone who feels desperate to lose weight quickly and who feels under a deadline to rethink the situation. You didn't put that weight on overnight and it's not going to come off overnight no matter how you feel about it, so you might as well choose a different feeling to have about the situation—desperation won't change things and will only keep you from enjoying the journey. Instead of focusing on six weeks from now try visualizing how you'll feel and look a year from now. You'll have a much greater shot at achieving your goal and astronomically greater chances of holding on to it once you get there.

Plus you just might have some unexpected fun on the ride along the way.

Week Six

Week Six: Journal

Keep writing. Feelings, impressions, thoughts, poetry quotes, food, exercise logs, favorite movies, CDs—I don't care. Rename the journal "The Story of Me" if you like.

This is a good time to remind you of the rule that you can't show it to anyone. One of the stumbling blocks some people seem to come up against when they use their journal regularly is curiosity from husbands, wives, lovers, friends and the like. "Hey, whatcha got in there?" they ask. "Writing anything about me?" If you tell them it's private, they'll often pout and say some version of the following: "Hey, if you're not writing anything negative in there, how come you won't let me see it?" The answer is simple: You gave your word. It's the rules. Tell them the program only works if you do it that way. Tell them whatever you want. Just know that you can't show it to them. If you even think, on some level, that someone else might see it, you will not treat it in the same way.

And by the way, it's only "the rules" because *you say so*, a distinction we'll be talking about a lot more in Chapter 15 ("Rewrite Your Story").

These rules go double for you if you are a professional writer, by the way. Journal writing was always particularly hard for me, because I had a little voice up there saying, "Hey, this stuff is pretty good, maybe you should publish it someday." *Wrong.* If you want to write professionally, keep your writing sketches somewhere else. Buy another journal, it's fine with me. But your Shape Up journal is for your eyes and yours alone.

Week Six: To-Do List

Two more things come off this week, but I won't tell if you want to up the ante. Hopefully, the to-do list is becoming a regular part of your life by now. It might be a good idea to start looking at some of the bigger things that have been taking up space in your brain, larger projects that you have always wanted to do, and begin to break them into smaller steps. Then start doing the smaller steps. It's the to-do list version of losing weight one pound at a time.

At one point in time, my wife, Cassandra, decided that she wanted to do a calendar featuring the women of daytime television with the proceeds going to charity. A much bigger project than you might imagine, and one on which it was very easy to procrastinate. Eventually she broke it down into groups of tasks: finding a charity, a hotel to host, a photographer, an airline, contacting the women, the sponsor, the finance and business people, and so on. Then she broke the groups down even further into to-do lists. Eventually the mini-chores on the lists became manageable, largely because they were broken down into concrete tasks: a phone call here, an e-mail there.

Interestingly, once she made the decision to take action (notice I didn't say anything about "commitment") and began the process of constructing the to-do lists, something very remarkable happened. She was approached by a very experienced businessman who was putting together an on-line store for soap opera stars; she met with him and eventually partnered with him on the project. The calendar, profits from which go to the Children's Miracle Foundation, is currently in development.

I can't prove this, but I can tell you that it's been my experience time and time again that once you begin to take actions toward a goal, no matter how small the actions may seem, a project kind of takes on a momentum and energy of its own and stuff starts to happen and fall into place. This is true whether it's making a calendar, making a movie, going back to school, buying a house, or losing a ton of weight.

The trick is to step off the start line.

Week Six: Developing Your Food Plan

If you haven't already begun to really monitor sugar intake, now's the time to do so. Pay attention to labels. Remember that by law they have to list ingredients by amount, so if you see sugar as the first or second ingredient that should be a red flag. Manufacturers are sneaky, though. They know that people know this, so they will often put several different kinds of sweetener into a product; this way, none of the ingredients by itself is contributing that much to the overall product, but taken together as a whole, these sugars are the major ingredient. Look for ingredients like fruit juice concentrate, high fructose corn syrup, barley malt, brown rice syrup, lactose, maltodextrin, maltose, or anything ending in "-itol" (mannitol, sorbitol, xylitol). Frightening, isn't it? For some people, cutting down on (or cutting out) sugar may just be one the most profound changes they can make to the diet and may reap the greatest benefits in terms of energy, mood fluctuations, and insulin levels.

Week Six: Exercise

Continue walking program with the following modification:

Twice a week, 45 minutes. Once a week 30 minutes. The remaining two days are weight training days—walk 20 minutes on those days.

To review, your program now looks like this:

Day One	Day Two	Day Three	Day Four	Day Five
walk 45 min.	walk 20 min. weight training	walk 30 min.	walk 20 min. weight training	walk 45 min.

On weight training days, you will now add this final exercise:

LATERAL RAISES (SHOULDERS)

Take a dumbbell in each hand and hold at the sides of your body, palms facing inward. Stand with feet-shoulder width apart, knees slightly bent. Don't lean backward (Figure 13.5).

Raise your arms up and out to the sides till they are parallel to the ground, or "crucifix" position (Figure 13.6), then lower back down. Repeat for 8–12 reps.

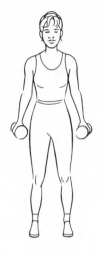

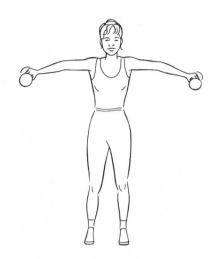

Fig. 13.5   Fig. 13.6

To review: Twice a week, for example, Monday and Friday, you walk for 45 minutes. Once a week, for example, Wednesday, you walk for 30. The other two days, for example, Tues and Thursday, you walk for twenty minutes and then perform one complete "circuit" of the seven weight training exercises, (one set each).

This is what it looks like:

Day One	Day Two	Day Three	Day Four	Day Five
walk 45 min.	walk 20 min.	walk 30 min.	walk 20 min.	walk 45 min.
	crunches		crunches	
	squats		squats	
	bench press		bench press	
	row		row	
	bicep curls		bicep curls	
	tricep dips		tricep dips	
	lateral raises		lateral raises	

End with a gentle stretch and relaxation.

Week Six: Self-Assessment Questionnaire

1. How much time, really, do you take to care for yourself? (Hint: Don't judge it, just tell it.)
2. What does "caring for yourself" mean to you? What does it look like?

THE MYTH OF MOTIVATION: "IT'S THE ACTION, STUPID!"

14

Every ball that comes to me is a decision.

— BILLIE JEAN KING, TENNIS LEGEND

Let me let you in on the big secret about motivation. And about its cousin, willpower: They're highly overrated. And you don't need either of them to be successful at losing weight.

I once had the pleasure of knowing Rob Kapilow, one of the great young conductors in America. In fact, when I was working as a professional musician, he was my teacher. One day, he told me that he had just been called by the Boston Opera Company to be a last minute replacement for an ailing conductor. He needed to conduct a Verdi opera (they're *very* long), which he was not familiar with. Not only that, it was in a language that he didn't speak fluently. Not only *that*, the conducting gig was in four days. He basically had a weekend to learn the piece.

By the way, the Boston Opera does not suffer fools gladly, if you get my drift.

Rob was completely sanguine.

I, on the other hand, was incredulous. "How are you ever going to learn this piece in time?" I asked. Already I was reeling from the sheer enormity of the task, the impossibility of it and the anxiety that would have to be associated with not only learning it under such pressure, but being able to lead some very curmudgeonly musicians in its performance.

"Simple," he said with a twinkle and a shrug. "I'll learn it the same way I learn any piece.

"One bar at a time."

That simple four-word statement taught me everything I ever needed to know about motivation and accomplishment.

See, it's not the task—getting in shape, losing forty (or a hundred) pounds—that's defeating you; it's your perception of it. You're being defeated by allowing yourself to feel the sheer "enormity" of the full opera, so to speak. That's exactly what most of us do when confronted with changing our bodies. What's interesting to me is that we often don't do it in other arenas of our lives. For example, if you decide to have a child, do you consider the huge task of the next eighteen years, from the number of hours it will take each day to nurse her and watch after her while she's an infant to the amount of money it will take to send her to college? If you went to university, did you look at the whole four years and think of the number of books you'd have to read, the amount of material you'd need to learn, the number of tests you'd have to pass in order to get that degree? Probably not. No, in both cases, though you might have glanced down the road at the bigger picture, you probably did the "day-to-dayness" of it one day at a time.

Or, in Rob's case, one bar at a time.

And if you are to be successful in your current goal—and you will be—you're going to have to do it the same way.

One pound at a time.

I have never, ever been a sports fan, don't follow a single team sport, never have, but I believe a sports analogy might be useful here. If you're not a sports fan either, stay with me, and if you are, you'll probably appreciate this even more than I do.

Let's say you're watching a big basketball game. Score's tied, stakes are high, it's the playoffs, almost the end of the fourth quarter, and Michael Jordan's got the ball and is about to take the shot. Quick, now, what do you think he's thinking?

Do you think he's thinking: Man, I gotta make this shot, because my team depends on it and if I don't we don't get to go the finals and then we don't win the championship and no one's gonna make as much dough on endorsements and everyone's counting on me?

Bah. Humbug. Too much chatter.

You know what he's thinking about?

He's thinking about how to get the ball into the hoop.

See, "motivation" doesn't have to be about keeping your eye on some distant goal, like winning a pennant, or finishing college, or losing a hundred pounds. "Motivation" is much more simple. It's being in the moment, making a decision *right now* about this thing in front of you. All the rest is chatter, and very unproductive chatter at that. When sports coaches talk about "choking" that's what they mean: *The chatter got in the way*. The pressure and all the "meaning" of what you're about to do or not do interfered with your ability to concentrate on what's in front of you. The best players are the ones who don't think about all that. They just look at the basket and concentrate on getting the ball in. Period. And that's what you've got to do with weight loss.

Every meal, every day for you is a chance to put the ball in the hoop.

Forget motivation, and forget willpower. The only thing you need is a plan for action. Motivation and willpower are concepts that live in your head, and you spend far too much time there already. We've been brainwashed into thinking that we need to understand a behavior thoroughly before we can change it. But let me tell you something—you can learn *emotions* from *actions*. It's not just a one-way street where you have to first *understand* where a fear is coming from before you can *do* something about it. The old psychotherapeutic maxim that understanding your behavior always leads to change is just not a good premise to operate on. First of all, it doesn't always happen that way, and second of all, even if it did, which it doesn't, you could get old and gray before you completely understood why you did something, and there would be absolutely no guarantee that you would change the thing you wanted to change in the first place. (People understand why they smoke, and it doesn't help them much to quit.) So understanding isn't much use, and neither, as we have seen, is willpower.

All you really need is action. All you really need is a plan for how to put one foot in front of the other. Don't worry about how you feel about it, and don't worry about if you understand it, and for goodness sake, don't worry about whether you have enough motivation to do it.

Each meal, each morsel of food, each exercise session is a *decision*, right then and there, about whether to take an action that furthers your goals or whether to do something that doesn't. Do you want to get the ball into the hoop? Right now? This minute? That's all you need to ask yourself. Thinking about the long range, and the consequences, and of what it all "means" about you as a person is just so much chatter in your mind. Get the ball into the hoop. This time. Now. And if it doesn't go in, the *next* time you get the ball, try again. You get to make that decision each and every time. That's the only "motivation" you need. Thinking about losing a hundred pounds (or ten or fifty) would be like Michael Jordan worrying about the endorsements and the playoffs and the post-game interviews when all he needs to worry about right now, in this moment, is how to get the ball to go through that little basket.

And by the way, another secret: Concentrating only on getting the ball into the hoop, each time the ball is in his hands, is *exactly* how he got to win all those championships and endorsements. You get those things by being a great player, and being a great player means thinking about nothing but getting the ball in the hoop every time the ball comes your way. You win at the weight loss game the same way: not by listening to all the chatter in your head about what will or will not happen, but by learning to master the single, everyday situations that present themselves in front of you.

You learn what to do with the ball. That's what this program is about. Getting the ball in the hoop. That's all the motivation you need. All the rest is just mental energy taking away from the concentration needed to sink the basket.

Postscript: What do you think Michael Jordan does on those occasions when he misses the basket? Do you think he thinks, "Man, missed that shot, what a drag, I suck, I've ruined everything, might as well not play this game, I'm a downer, I've let the team down, there go the playoffs and the endorsments . . ."

Nope. Here's what happens:

He forgets about it and starts all over and the next time he's got the ball he thinks about one thing and one thing only: getting it in the basket.

To lose weight successfully, you must learn the Rob Kapilow (and the Michael Jordan) lesson. Whether it's studying music, losing weight, shooting baskets or building sobriety, the message is the same and you ignore it at your own peril.

How do you lose weight successfully?

Simple.

One pound at a time.

REWRITE YOUR STORY 15

The past does not equal the future.

—TONY ROBBINS

Sex appeal is 50 percent what you've got,
and 50 percent what people *think* you've got.

—SOPHIA LOREN

Sex appeal is 100 percent
what *you* think you've got.

—JONNY BOWDEN

This chapter is the most important chapter in the entire Shape Up program. If you really *get* what I'm about to tell you, and I mean really, really *get* it, you can change your life.

No kidding.

Everything in life that has ever happened to you, from the smallest encounter with the grocery clerk to the most meaningful event in your personal life story, can be broken down into two components: The first is "what happened." The second is "what you think it means." The problem is most of us think they are the same thing.

They're not.

Let's say an actress goes to an audition, spends thirty seconds in the room with the director and is told "Thank you very much." She leaves the audition thinking she did a terrible job, she has no talent, she will never get anywhere in this business, she ought to give up the profession, she's getting too old to get hired, and maybe her mother was right and she ought to get a real job. (If you think this doesn't happen on a daily basis, I respectfully submit that you don't know actors!) "What happened" is that she went to an audition and spent thirty seconds in the room. All the rest is "story," a story that she made up. That story may or may not be true. (It is *probably*

175

not, but it doesn't matter. Woody Allen, for example, rarely spends any time with actors in the audition room because it makes him uncomfortable, and he only brings them in for a minute to see what they look like in person. Other directors make a split second decision that they *like* the actor and are going to call her back anyway, so they spend virtually no time with her the first time around.) In any event, whether what you made up is true or not, your *experience* of the event comes not from "what happened" but from the *story* you made up about it. Your take-away experience comes from the *meaning* you gave to the event, not from the event itself. What we make an experience mean is something that is completely our own creation. But we rarely see this. We deny our power to *create* experience, thinking instead that experience is something that "happens" to us.

Let's say I lose the lease on my apartment, which I happen to like very much. I have a number of choices about what to make this "mean," but I'll give you two. Story number one: "*Oh my God, I lost my apartment. I'll have nowhere to live. Where will I ever find another one at such a great price? I'm going to have to go on welfare. My world is ending!*" Or . . . "What an opportunity to find some new space and get rid of some old junk. I get to re-invent myself and my surroundings. Let's party!" See, both are "stories." "What happened" is that I lost my apartment. All the rest of it is made up. And guess who gets to make it up? Guess who gets to write the story?

You got it.

Suppose you gained five pounds (or one hundred). Story: I'm a useless, unmotivated jerk. I'll never lose weight. I'm a big loser. I'll never be attractive, be sexy, find a mate, be a winner—pick anything you like. Sound familiar? The real truth is: *You gained five pounds* (or a *hundred*). Period. It doesn't *mean* anything. All the rest is stuff you make up. That's the punch line, folks. It's stuff you make up! You *and only you* get to author the story.

Want a great example of the difference a story can make in the way you experience the world (and the way the world experiences *you*)? Imagine that I'm a short girl from the Bronx with large thighs and hips and a big butt. (And, by the way, I want to be a movie star.) That's "what happened." That's "*what is.*" Now here's story number one (the most popular choice): "*I don't look like any of the models in the magazine or any of the actresses in Hollywood. I'll never be considered pretty. I'll never be attractive. No one will ever like this look. I must lose weight or no one will ever think I'm sexy. What's the point? I have fat thighs and hips and butt and I'm ethnic and short and I'll never look like Gwyneth Paltrow.*"

Here's story number two: "I have a big butt and I think it's the sexiest thing on two wheels. Think I'll just go on and flaunt it." (And by the way, because *I* really believe it, the whole world is going to believe it too. I'll just single-handedly change the standard of what sexy "looks" like.)

By the way, my name is Jennifer Lopez.

You make it up! The only thing that was "so" about Jennifer Lopez's looks was that she had a bigger butt than any actress in Hollywood. But she chose to make that *mean* something entirely different than most people would have chosen—yes, *chosen*—to make it mean. The story she made up about it *empowered* her instead of diminished her. Since *you're* the one who makes up your own story, why not make one up that empowers *you*?

Remember, weight is just a number. If it defeats you, if it discourages you, if it destroys you, it's only because *you're* making it *mean* something. You're making up a story about it that does not serve you. So how about making up one that does serve you? Since you make it up anyway, why not make up one that supports you instead of defeats you? How about rewriting that story? I know, I know, you're going to tell me that everyone else agrees with your story, but *so what*? Everyone in the world *agreed* that Jennifer Lopez had too big a butt to be a Hollywood star and that Barbra Streisand had too big a nose. And don't ever bother asking Cindy Crawford how many people told her that her career was history unless she got that ugly "thing" taken off her upper lip.

Your happiness or lack thereof is *not* contained in what happens. It's a function of what you make it *mean*. It's the story you tell *about* what happened, both to yourself and to the world. I'm going to give you an exercise, right now, to help you change how you do that. I'm going to help you develop the skill to write stories that are filled with opportunity and possibility. And all you have to do is say two words:

So what?

When you feel yourself getting discouraged over something in your life—anything at all, your weight, your job, your relationship, a fight with your boss, a broken computer, you name it—I want you to try the following exercise: Say what it is that happened. And then ask, "So what?"

And tell yourself the answer.

When you've done that, ask the question again.

Now I don't want you to ask this in the same spirit as you would ask, "*Who cares?*" This exercise is *not* about "who cares?" and it's certainly not about "whatever . . ." This exercise is about *you* finding out what *you* made something mean. About getting to the bottom of what frightens you, makes you feel bad, disempowers or defeats you. This exercise is about lightening the load. It's about finding the opportunity. It's about turning the corner and seeing *possibility* rather than closed doors and dead ends.

If you think you can't do it, if you think "what happened" is so bad that there simply is *no other way to experience it* than the way you experience it, consider this: I have had people on my talk show that have looked right in the face of some of the most horrific events you can imagine. Cancer. Death of a child. Rape. And have asked, in their own way, "And soooo . . . ?" They have looked inside themselves to see what possibilities were contained in that experience. They've taken it apart and put it back together, and in the process discovered something deeply profound about their own power.

Let's take one of the worst cases possible. "*I have cancer.*" And sooooooooo? "*Well, I might die.*" And soooooooo? "*Well, I might never get to tell the people I love what they mean to me, or make a difference in the world.*" Aha! Now we're getting somewhere. I don't care if you have ten minutes left on the planet, there is still some realm in which you have choice. And the discovery of that fact is the most empowering realization you're ever likely to make in this life. If there are people on the planet who have created opportunities for growth and expansion and personal power out of tumors growing on the outside of their chest—*and there are*—then what could you create right here, right now?

Terry McDonald is a New York cop who, at the age of twenty-eight, with two small children and a third on the way, was shot during a brutal gunfight. The bullet lodged in his spine. He's now a paraplegic. That's "what happened." Some time ago, he forgave his attacker. When last heard from he was headed across Ireland in a wheelchair, pushed by volunteers, on a mission to spread peace and teach reconciliation to two sides who had been mortal enemies for the better part of a century.

Asking "So what?" does not mean that you don't care about life and that nothing matters. In fact, it's just the opposite. It doesn't mean there isn't great stuff and terrible stuff out there. It just means you don't sit there and passively let life happen to you. You are the person who writes the book about what it is all going to mean. This exercise is about one thing and one thing only: breaking the "glue" between a "fact" and a "story." The "story" is the thing you make up about the fact, the thing you make it mean. The "so what?" exercise is a way of owning your authorship of this story.

Once you break "what happened" (what *is*) away from *what you make it mean*, you have a brilliant opportunity. You can rewrite the story that you made up in the first place.

If Terry McDonald could do it with a paralyzing gunshot wound, mere mortals like you and me can surely do it with the scale.

Cellulite

Cellulite is fat that has been trapped in fibrous pockets close to the skin. Like water in very shallow, shaded creeks, it tends to stay put even when the rest of the river is drying up. Some people have put forth the theory that cellulite is a particular kind of fat, with a higher level of toxins stored in it, but this is pure armchair speculation.

It may help to think of cellulite and saddlebags (or any pockets of stubborn fat that don't seem to respond to anything you do) like plaque below the gum line in the mouth. It seems that when there are little pockets around the gum line, bacteria and plaque get in there and they are devilishly hard to get out once they've taken up residence. No matter how well you brush your teeth, once they're in there, they're in there and surface cleaning just won't dislodge them. It may well be the same sort of situation with cellulite and saddlebags.

Now is there any *good* news about this? Well, yes, maybe there is.

I think we can reasonably assume that many processes in the body, including fat breakdown and detoxification in general, could be slowed down or otherwise interfered with by food sensitivities, food allergies, less than perfect digestion and absorption or a poor diet. So is it prudent to try the caveman approach to eating, removing as much as possible of the modern day processed and manufactured food products? I think so. In fact, the best thing you can do for stubborn (and even not-so-stubborn) pockets of fat is to try a diet as absolutely free of possible allergens, processed and refined foods, sugar and other problem food "products" as possible. You might even try temporarily removing some of the more recent arrivals on the nutritional evolutionary scene, like wheat and dairy and soy, just to see what happens.

Will a caveman diet, coupled with the best exercise program you can manage, done consistently, remove saddlebags or cellulite? Honestly, I don't know. But I do know that short of liposuction, it has the best chance of success and is probably the only path you can take that might actually work.

Oh, and one more thing. I want to let you in on a little secret.

I've been a male for—well, a number of decades. During that time I have had my share of locker room discussions, "over drinks" discussions, "what should I do about this girl" discussions. I have spoken to probably thousands of other males in my lifetime, and many of those discussions were about females. I have overheard thousands more conversations, virtually all of them out of the listening range of female ears and therefore—it's probably safe to say—representative of what men really think. That said, I'm going to let you in on a secret. I think it's time you should know this. Listen carefully, because it's a very important piece of information and you may be hearing it for the first time. You may even find it hard to believe, but let me assure you that it's true.

In all that time, in all those conversations, I never *once* heard a man complain about cellulite on a woman. Not one single time. I know this statement is not based on a scientific study, but I'll stand by it nonetheless. It's a pretty good clinical observation based on a lot of living as a male. I truly, truly believe that cellulite is a far more important concept for women than it is for men and that, quite frankly, along with stretch marks, men just don't really care about it nearly as much as you think they do.

Just thought you ought to know.

WEEKS SEVEN AND EIGHT 16

Week Seven

Week Seven: Journal

I want you to play the "so what?" exercise with the facts of your life, and I want you to write down what you find out. Take any experience, any feeling, any event and ask yourself, "What happened?" Don't editorialize, don't judge, don't talk about what *should* have been, don't elaborate. Just say *what happened*. As the detective on the old TV series used to say, "Just the facts, ma'am, just the facts." It can be something that happened, or something that is so right now. Keep it short and simple. If this is hard to do, notice that. Notice how much "story" wants to creep in, even in the simple telling of what happened, even when the assignment is to *not* tell a story. (If you're noticing this, you're on your way to a breakthrough.)

When you've finished writing "what happened," or stating "what's so," ask yourself "*So what?*" Write down everything you made that particular "what happened" *mean*. Be very specific. All the ramifications, everything you think follows from it, everything you think is *inseparable* from it, how you feel about it. Take yourself down the whole road you paved for yourself. Follow every nook and cranny. Did "what happened" cause your experience, or was it *what you told yourself was true about what happened?* Start making the distinction.

Now make up a different story. I don't care how hard this is, and for many people it'll be really, really hard. Do it anyway. A little voice is going to tell you there is no other story that could be told out of "what happened." The little voice is lying. Make one up anyway. Then make up another.

When you're done, make up one more.

Notice anything getting lighter?

If you *didn't* notice it getting lighter, what did you make *that* mean?

Just keep looking. And keep telling the truth about what you're seeing. When you're done, look some more.

(Psst. . . . Are you making this mean something very serious?)

Week Seven: To-Do List

Take a look at a couple of things on your to-do list. What stories did you make up about them? What did you make it mean if you did do them? What did you make it mean if you *didn't* do them? So what?

Do a couple more things on your to-do list. (Or don't.) Notice what you make that mean.

Are you beginning to get the joke?

Keep looking.

Week Seven: Developing Your Food Plan

It's time to begin to ask yourself some questions about the *quality* of what you're eating. How closely does your food resemble the form in which it would be found in nature? If you're eating meat, how processed is it? Are your eggs from free range chickens? Does the majority of the food you're eating come without a label? Are you eating at least some raw foods each day? Are you beginning to balance how much nutrition and energy is in the food you eat against how convenient it is? Is the balance beginning to shift?

Make your own personal check list of foods that sustain and nourish you. See how many of them you can include on a daily basis.

Week Seven: Exercise

Now it's time to really up the ante. Two big modifications this week:

- Walking: Go for 45 minutes three days a week, and 30 minutes on weight training days.
- Weight training: Go through the full circuit of seven exercises and then repeat it for a total of two complete circuits.

A "circuit" is defined as a complete set of the seven exercises, one set per exercise. Try to move from one exercise to the next with minimum rest in between.

Here's how it looks:

Day One	Day Two	Day Three	Day Four	Day Five
walk 45 min.	walk 30 min.	walk 45 min.	walk 30 min.	walk 45 min.
	First Circuit		**First Circuit**	
	crunches		crunches	
	squats		squats	
	bench press		bench press	
	row		row	
	bicep curls		bicep curls	
	tricep dips		tricep dips	
	lateral raises		lateral raises	
	Second Circuit		**Second Circuit**	
	crunches		crunches	
	squats		squats	
	bench press		bench press	
	row		row	
	bicep curls		bicep curls	
	tricep dips		tricep dips	
	lateral raises		lateral raises	

Week Seven: Self-Assessment Questionnaire

1. What does your weight "say" about you?
2. Do *you* say that or does your weight? Who made that up? (Helpful hint: If you think "someone else" or "society" made it up, how much do you agree with it? Who made *that* story up?)

Week Eight

Week Eight: Journal

Think of someone you know in your life who is a procrastinator. Maybe it's you, or at least maybe it was you before you began this book. Now write down what being a procrastinator *means*. What do you know about a person who is a procrastinator? What's so about him? Take a minute and jot down what comes to mind before reading further.

Good. Did you say people who procrastinate are lazy? Unmotivated? Fearful of success? Irresponsible? Come on, fess up.

Now I'm going to tell you something. Procrastinators are wise. They take time to evaluate. They are thinkers and seekers. They're romantic dreamers. They take longer to get stuff done, but so what? They're also more likely to come up with far more creative stuff than the average person when they finally do get around to taking action.

Now I'm going to tell you one more thing. *I just made that up.* Just like *you* made up that the procrastinator is lazy and unmotivated. Neither story is any more "true" than the other.

And you know what else? Being a procrastinator—or being fat, or being tall, or being beautiful, or having one leg or winning the French Open or breaking up with a lover—doesn't mean anything except what *you say it means.*

Beginning to get the point?

Week Eight: To-Do List

Make up an assignment for the to-do list. Give your word that you're going to do that assignment. Your commitment to keep your word only matters because *you say it does.*

Week Eight: Developing Your Food Plan

It's been my experience that people are in very different places with their food plans by the time we get to the eighth week. Remember that our goal is to discover what works and tell the truth about it. For most people, what works is going to be some combination of high-quality protein, traditional and nourishing fats, vegetables and fruits, and perhaps limited amounts of low-sugar, high-fiber starches like oatmeal and sweet potatoes and beans. The exact amounts and proportions are going to ultimately have to be your own design, but by now you have everything you need to craft a food plan that honors the unique needs of your body. Remember once again that losing weight is a process, not an event.

When something gets in the way, look it in the eye, tell the truth about it, disarm it and move on.

And, as Winston Churchill said in his address to the graduating class of Oxford University:

"*Never, never, ever give up.*"

Week Eight: Exercise

Continue with the walking program but up it to 45 minutes a day, even on weight training days. On weight training days, continue to do two full circuits of the seven exercises.

It looks like this:

Day One	Day Two	Day Three	Day Four	Day Five
walk 45 min.	walk 45 min.	walk 45 min.	walk 45 min.	walk 45 min.
	First Circuit		**First Circuit**	
	crunches		crunches	
	squats		squats	
	bench press		bench press	
	row		row	
	bicep curls		bicep curls	
	tricep dips		tricep dips	
	lateral raises		lateral raises	
	Second Circuit		**Second Circuit**	
	crunches		crunches	
	squats		squats	
	bench press		bench press	
	row		row	
	bicep curls		bicep curls	
	tricep dips		tricep dips	
	lateral raises		lateral raises	

OK, that's really it. This is the core of a wonderful program that can keep you healthy, fit and lean for a very, very long time. If you haven't been able to quite do it yet, trust me, you will. Just keep showing up.

And when you're ready to move on, there's a lot of ways to do it. Here are just some of them:

- Turn the walks into jogs, or do walk/jogs, alternating between the two till you're able to go the distance.
- Do interval training on the walk (walk/jog) days. What that means is you go real fast—whatever that is for you—for about a minute, then bring the intensity (and your heart rate) back down while you walk (or jog slower) for a few minutes (that's called the "recovery"). Then repeat. You can do three to ten intervals in a given training session, and if you need to make it harder still, you can always extend the time of the fast interval and decrease the time of the recovery.
- Add more weight to the weight training exercises.
- Add more repetitions to the weight training exercises.
- Add another circuit to the weight training day.
- Add more exercises to the circuit (by the time you're ready to do this one, believe me, you'll have found all *kinds* of resources from which to learn new exercises—other exercisers, trainers, videos, the Internet, your local gym).
- Change the circuit routine by substituting some of the new exercises that you'll find (see above paragraph), just for variety. You *are* allowed to have fun doing this, you know.
- Mix and match the "cardio" (walk/jog) part of your workout with the weight training part. Go for a fifteen minute walk/jog, then do a circuit. Do cardio another fifteen minutes before doing the second circuit. The combinations are endless.
- If you're keeping records, it might be interesting for you to go back now and see what you were doing in the very beginning. Think about how hard it was to do the workout even in the first or second week, and look at what you're doing now. Inspiring, isn't it? But if by chance your own pace has been a little slower—OK *a lot* slower—than the pacing of the book, who cares? That's fine too. Remember, *getting in shape is a process, not an event.*

Week Eight: Self-Assessment Questionnaire

1. What would you most like to be remembered for?
2. What would you most like people to say about you?
3. What are you doing to make that happen?

BEING IS BELIEVING 17

Years ago, I had one of the greatest teachers on the planet, who I'm sure would want to remain nameless for the purposes of this story but would nonetheless get a big kick out of my telling it in this context. The teacher had developed an enormous, almost cult-like following, and people were willing to go almost anywhere to hear him speak. One day, he was scheduled to give a talk at the old Cow Palace in San Francisco, an enormous stadium-type venue in the heart of the city. Unfortunately, the talk was scheduled around the same time that the news was predicting an earthquake.

Nonetheless, people flocked to the Cow Palace to hear the teacher, a fact that left the media somewhat stunned. So they interviewed him. "Teacher," they said, "how is it that people are leaving the city in droves, but thousands of people are driving *in* to hear you speak at the Cow Palace? Everyone is afraid of the earthquake, yet you've managed to sell out the biggest auditorium in San Francisco on a night when people can't get out of here fast enough!" "Simple," said the teacher, smiling. "I've decided there isn't going to be an earthquake. There just isn't going to be an earthquake, so there's nothing to worry about." The reporters looked around at each other as if to say, *This guy is crazy.* Just before walking away from the stunned reporters, the teacher looked around and said, with a twinkle in his eye, "So don't forget—there's not gonna be an earthquake . . . but if you hear the earth rumble, you'll know I changed my mind."

What is, is. What isn't, isn't. You have two choices: Choose it or don't. Choosing "what is" doesn't mean that you blindly accept whatever happens and that you don't care about it. Choosing what's so simply lets you practice your ability to create your own experience. Choosing *what is* gives you space to make something else happen. If you're one hundred pounds right now, or five hundred pounds, *choose that* and move on. Believe me, right now, or at any given moment in time, you're not going to change the number of pounds you are *in that second.* So you have only one choice in *any given moment*—choose what is, or yell at it. One option creates space, one creates resistance. Which would you rather have? Tell the truth about what is, preferably without volumes of "story." Resisting what's so simply makes it persist. Choose it and be with it and you can move on.

This, by the way, is very different than "positive thinking." For example, let's say I weigh three hundred pounds, and I hate the way I look. Here are some examples of how I could tell the truth about what's so right now *in this moment.*

- I weigh three hundred pounds.
- I'm angry right now.
- It's Tuesday.
- The sun is out.
- It's 5:05 P.M.

That's "what's so." Period. Say it, choose it, and move on. Believe me, everything else is chatter and is much more likely to defeat you than to support you in creating something new. When you tell the truth about something and choose *what is* in the moment that it's so, you lighten up— and when you lighten up many things will seem possible that would just not happen in any other state of mind.

Life—and weight loss—are just giant games of Chutes and Ladders. You land where you land and you choose it and move on. Just keep showing up.

Because the action is *not* in always avoiding the chutes.

The action is about staying in the game.

IT'S A WAR OUT THERE 18

Metabolism, Emotions, Family and Other Pitfalls

I don't deserve this award, but I have
arthritis, and I don't deserve that either.

— JACK BENNY

"What More Do You Want From Me?"

"I just can't lose weight, no matter what I do."

"I've tried everything."

"I'm working out three times a week and watching what I eat, and still nothing happens."

The frustration that people experience when they feel they're making changes in their diet and yet nothing is happening with their weight is a big stumbling block to progress. Every day I hear some version of the following refrain: "No matter what I do, the weight won't come off."

OK, I won't lie to you. Losing weight is one of the most difficult things in the world to do. Anyone who tells you it's easy, effortless or mindless is lying; anyone who tells you they have a system that lets you eat all you want, make no changes in your life, lose weight while you sleep, or lose weight just by breathing (yes, I actually saw an infomercial hawking that one) should be trusted about as much as a used-car salesman at an annual going-out-of-business sale.

So why, if it's so impossible, are we even bothering to talk about it?

Well, I didn't say it was *impossible*. I said it was *difficult*. I said the odds were against you. But you know what? The same is true in many of life's arenas. It's true in the acting profession. It's true in professional sports. It's true in the world of Internet start-ups. Yet every year New York City and Los Angeles are flooded with aspiring actors, every day some young entrepreneur is maxing out her credit cards to start a business, and every season thousands of high school hopefuls try to get the attention of a big-league scout.

And you know what?

Some of them are going to make it.

Against overwhelming odds, every year there are major success stories. Some of those aspiring actors who are now waiting tables actually *do* become stars. Some of those unpublished manuscripts *do* become best-sellers. Some of those high school hopefuls *do* actually go on to seven fig-ure big league contracts. Some of those Internet start-ups *will* change the way we do business in America.

And some people *will* lose weight and keep it off.

And you can be one of them.

But you *can't* do it by accident, and you *can't* do it while you sleep, and you *can't* do it "easily and effortlessly," because if it were possible to do that, no one would be fat.

And you have a much better chance if you know, *really know*, what you're up against. If you have no illusions, have your eyes wide open and have absolutely no misconceptions about what you're going to confront. But if you're willing to roll up your sleeves and really—I mean *really*—understand the enemy, well then, there is no reason you can't be one of the ones who make it.

And make no mistake. It is a war out there.

I've had people tell me that they've tried everything, that they've made really good changes in their eating (though what many of those people consider to be "good" changes doesn't always match what I consider to be good changes, as you've learned), that they're now exercising a few times a week, yet nothing is happening. The scale is not budging. In some cases, it's even going up. They're beginning to feel like nothing they do can pos-sibly make a difference.

At that point, I ask the following question: "If I put you in marine boot camp right now, with an exercise regime that would challenge Demi Moore in *G.I. Jane*, and a twelve-hundred-calorie-a-day diet with absolute-ly no refined foods or sugar and adequate amounts of protein and fat, and I kept you in that boot camp for one year, do you think you'd look exact-ly the same after a year as you do now?" And once they say "No, of course not," I tell them the following old joke.

"Would you go to bed with me for ten million dollars?" asks the elderly gen-tleman of the young socialite. She thinks about it a minute. "Ten million dollars?" she asks. "Yup," he replies. "OK, I'll do it." "Great," he says. "How about for ten dollars?" She furiously slaps his face and storms out of the room, saying, "What do you think I am?" "Madam," the gentleman replies, "we've already established that. Now we're simply negotiating a price."

Look, if you agree that you'd lose weight and that your body would change significantly on the boot camp regimen I described a couple of paragraphs earlier, then we've already established something: *You can lose weight.* It *can* be done. Now we're just going to negotiate what you have to do to make it happen.

And this is where it gets tricky.

Look, some people can lose weight simply by cutting out dessert. Some people need to go to boot camp. Most people are somewhere in-between those two extremes. Problem is, everyone wants to believe they are closer to the "just cut out dessert and walk a little" end of the spectrum. Unfortunately, more of us fall closer to the "need to go to *G.I. Jane* camp" part of the curve.

Am I saying you have to go to *G.I. Jane* extremes? No. But I'm saying that losing weight and staying in shape for most people takes a lot more than cutting out dessert and moderate exercise a few times a week. Will doing just a little make you healthier? You bet it will. Is it a step in the right direction? Absolutely. Should you be commended for taking those steps? Without a doubt. But this whole program is about telling the truth, especially to yourself. So let's tell the truth about this. If you've had a stubborn weight problem all your life, you're *not* going to lose serious weight and make *big* changes in your body unless you're willing to make *serious* changes.

And that means dealing with that little voice in your head that's yelling, "What more do you *want* from me? Haven't I done *enough*?"

I did tell you early on in the book that there was one exception to this "don't count calories" guideline, and that's what we're going to talk about right now. Every so often, a person will follow the healthy eating guidelines of the Shape Up program and . . . nothing happens. They almost always report feeling better, stronger, healthier—nothing to sneeze at, by the way—and sometimes even report that their clothes fit better, but the scale just doesn't seem to move even though they're doing all the right stuff. In cases like this, I often recommend calorie counting *as a temporary strategy.*

Maybe you're now eating all the right food but you're just eating too much of it. In cases like this, putting the food under the microscope, temporarily, can be a very useful strategy for finding "hidden" calories or for ferreting out a clearer picture of just how much food *you* really need to maintain *your* weight and how much needs to be cut to stimulate weight loss. No it's not fun, and no, it's not fair, but when you're doing everything else right and nothing is working, it's the way to go. Studies have consistently found that most people, even the best intentioned and most honest, underestimate the total amount of calories they take in on a regular basis. Maybe you don't count those delicious Frappaccinos you have once a day. Maybe you forgot about the taco chips you munched on before dinner came. Maybe you weren't as good a judge of what four (or five, or six) ounces looked like as you thought you were. Maybe, like many people, you didn't count the calories you drink. This kind of attention to detail, annoying as it is to most people, and resisted as it is by almost everyone, invariably reveals information that can make or break a weight loss plan.

Susan had a typical scenario. A writer, she lived an essentially sedentary life and had pretty much eaten anything she liked without thinking about it much. She had always battled a weight problem but in her thirties found herself seriously overweight and frightened about the possibility of diabetes. Determined to do something about it once and for all, she entered a weight loss program and began working out with a trainer twice a week. Although it was a painstaking process, over the course of a year she lost an admirable thirty pounds.

And then . . . her weight loss stalled. Wouldn't budge. Nada. Zilch. Zero.

Now here's the thing: That is not necessarily a bad place to be. Thirty pounds is a respectable amount of weight to lose. Susan had really accomplished something special and was to be completely and utterly congratulated on what she'd done, but she had reached a point that most weight loss books just don't talk much about. I call it the "choice point." It's the point when your body has adapted to the changes you've made in your life, and you can either choose to accept that and feel good about it, or not. As you may have learned by now: *How good you feel about your body is rarely a result of just the number of pounds you've lost.* Susan was entitled to feel pretty darn good about her thirty-pound weight loss.

But she didn't. She wanted more. Frustrated, she told me of her plight. She had made some good lifestyle changes. She was eating better. She was exercising for the first time. She felt like she had done everything she was "supposed" to do. But you know what?

For her body, for her metabolism, it just plain simply wasn't enough.

She had reached a "choice point," and she chose to continue losing weight. I suggested that she roll up her sleeves and begin keeping a detailed record of what she was eating and drinking. I wanted to know the percentage of her diet coming from protein, fat and carbohydrates on a meal-to-meal basis, and I wanted to know her exact caloric intake. And I wanted to know exactly how much she was exercising.

She didn't want to do that. I asked her why not.

"Well, for one thing that seems too much like dieting to me. 'Diet' implies you eat a certain way for a while, and maybe it works, but then you go back to the way you were eating before, and you regain all the weight. Counting calories implies restriction and deprivation. I want to make lifestyle changes, but I don't want to diet."

On the surface of it, Susan's explanation sounds like a very healthy and enlightened way to look at things. But in fact, it actually illustrates beautifully a big stumbling block that, if cleared up, could help her break through her plateau.

And the stumbling block is that deep-rooted feeling, not always articulated or even conscious, that voice in your head that's basically screaming, *"What more do you want from me?"*

Virtually everyone who has made positive changes in their life and doesn't see enough of the results they want to see suffers from the effect of this voice. You've never exercised in your life, and now you're making yourself do it two or three times a week. You always ate anything you felt like, now you've given up pizza and doughnuts. You went to a wedding and instead of eating four of everything, you watched what you ate. You only ate one dessert. And yet it's not happening. Your progress is stalled.

This is the point where people start thinking about giving up. They start thinking it's their metabolism. They begin thinking it's their genetic fate to be fat.

Well, let's make one thing about metabolism perfectly clear right now: *It isn't fair.* See, some people are wired in such a way that their bodies are just very forgiving of any cheating; they appear to be able to eat virtually anything they want and not gain weight. We all know people like that and we all hate them. Their tolerance for eating more than they should, or for eating the wrong things, is pretty wide. Maybe one day it will all catch up with them and they will pay for their transgressions, but right now, at least as far as food goes, they can get away with murder. On the other extreme there are those whose bodies have virtually a zero tolerance policy for the wrong kind of food choices. They glance sideways at a pint of Häagen-Dazs and their hips spontaneously grow an inch. If they're going to lose weight and keep it off, they simply cannot cheat.

As a kid I was always getting into trouble in school for the smallest infractions. It just seemed to be my fate. I had that "get into trouble" gene. Yet there was a kid in my class named Al Jaimeson who did stuff a hundred times worse than I did yet never seemed to get caught, and if he *did* get caught, he would escape with little more than a slap on the wrist. I would be two minutes late for class, he would play hooky for the day. I would whisper to my neighbor during silent period, he would shout obscenities from the school bus. I would throw a ball onto the neighbor's lawn, he would break their window. Yet I was always getting called into the principal's office, and Al was always getting off scot-free. One day, in a state of indignant rage as I was being given my umpteenth detention for some minor offense, I protested to my teacher, "*But what about Al Jaimeson?*" To which the teacher calmly replied, "What about him? Al is Al, and you are you."

Now, I know what I was thinking back then, and I know exactly what you're thinking right now: *It's not fair.* And you know what? You're absolutely right. It's not. But you know what else? Like it or not, *that's the way it is.*

Take gravity for example. Gravity isn't fair either. It just *is.* Gravity doesn't really care much whether you like it or not, or whether you agree with it or not. Try and work against gravity, try and fly up the down staircase, and guess what. You fall on your butt. Gravity doesn't care about fairness. Gravity just goes on being gravity. Metabolism is just metabolism. But you know what else? Once you *know* that, and understand and accept it, you can work with it. If you know the rules of gravity, you can have a very fine life, thank you very much, and you can walk, run, sail or even fly, because you know the rules, you know how it works, and you harness this action to work with you, in the service of your goals, instead of railing at the unfairness of it all while you continually land on your ass.

So, yes, metabolism isn't fair. Some people get fat by looking at some ice cream and some can eat anything they want and not gain a pound, but that is the luck of the genetic draw. It's not the particular roll of the dice that ultimately matters. It's how you play the number that comes up that makes you a winner or a loser, both in the weight loss game and in life. Armed with the information you need about how *your* body happens to work—not how it *should* work, or how you'd *like* it to work, but how it *does* work—you can make your life be the way you want it to.

Think: Backgammon. A game that is the perfect metaphor for weight loss. It combines luck and skill in a perfect mix that in many ways mirrors life itself. In backgammon, you throw a pair of dice—and how they land is completely a matter of luck, something over which you have no control. Yet the throw of the dice is just the beginning. How you play the move is what separates the great players from the amateurs. Great players can have real bad luck with the numbers that come up on their dice, but still wind up winners. Skill will win out over luck every single time.

So metabolism isn't fair. Make your peace with that right now. You may have made wonderful, terrific changes in the right direction, but you

know what? Your physiology does not give a you-know-what! Your physiology isn't making judgments on how hard or easy it is for you, it's not
giving you points for being good, it's not rewarding you with weight loss
because you tried so hard—it's just dealing with what you're eating and
doing with it what it was designed to do.

The *New Yorker* magazine doesn't care how long it takes you to write
a poem, or how hard it was for you to write a short story—it only cares
about whether it's good enough to publish. Some writers knock it out in
ten minutes and some take ten years. Who cares? It's the result that matters. I've known a lot of actresses in my time, and I'll tell you this: The
movie company doesn't give the role to the actress who studied the
longest and the hardest—they give it to the one who gives the best audition. Some actresses need to work their butts off to give a good audition
and some can just glance at the script and knock it out cold. *And it's the
same thing with your physiology.* Your body *does not care* how "hard" it is
for you, or how "good" you're being, it only deals with the end result,
which is what goes into your mouth and through your digestive system.
You may feel that the wedding buffet you recently attended was a great
triumph for you because you only ate one dessert and didn't have second portions of anything, but your physiology may still see what you
did eat as far more than you *needed* to eat. I know that's painful to hear,
but it's true. And until we really, really begin to look at what's coming
in—not only the calories, but the amounts of protein, fat and carbohydrates, on a daily basis—we have no way of defining our own personal
limits.

In other words: You must tell the truth about what *is* if you're going to
change things.

A well-known financial consultant and "life coach" in New York City,
Stephen Pollan, often speaks to clients about money and budget issues,
and one of the first things he has people do is keep scrupulous records of
how much cash they withdraw from the automatic teller machine during
the week, and where they spend it. People go nuts when they're told they
have to do this. They resist it passionately. And they resist it for the same
reason we resist keeping track of our food, or our calories. Money and
food are things about which it is simply more comfortable to be unconscious. But listen to me: It is virtually impossible to manage your money
if you don't know where it's going. If you're rich enough that those daily
cash withdrawals just fall into the category of "petty cash" and don't
impact your bottom line in any way, well then great, but for most people,
consciousness of where this money goes is a big step towards getting
finances in order.

And, yup, people hate keeping track. It's uncomfortable, it's not fun and it forces you to shine a harsh light on an area of your life that is normally pleasurable and that you don't want to examine too carefully. But make no mistake, it's a war out there, and if you want to play to win you need to know what you're up against. Our society is not set up to support healthy eating. If you're going to make serious changes, you need to start thinking like a warrior.

The True Warrior Creed: Know Thine Enemy!

Imagine this: a small village in a South American town. For centuries, the natives have gathered before going to work to chew on the coca plant. Cocaine is a major industry. It's available everywhere and an accepted part of social life. There are afternoon cocaine breaks. Employers make it readily available, as it increases productivity and keeps workers energized. It's a major player at social gatherings, communal and family events, an accompaniment to virtually every ritual of social life. Now: does this acceptability make cocaine any less dangerous or addictive? What would it be like for a villager in that mythical town to try to kick the habit?

Or consider tobacco. While it's no longer true here in America, cigarette smoking is a huge part of social life in other parts of the world. In Japan, there are cigarette machines on every corner. Advertisements for cigarettes abound and are found everywhere from subway trains to magazines to television. There are no such things as non-smoking restaurants. It's rare to find a Japanese salaryman in downtown Tokyo who isn't chain smoking throughout the business day. Are the Japanese any more protected from lung cancer than we are simply because smoking in Japan is a completely accepted part of life?

If you live in an industrial first-world nation like the United States, make no mistake about it: You are living with a toxic food supply. There's no beating around the bush here. It's as toxic and destructive to your health as cocaine is in the South American village and as cigarettes are in downtown Tokyo and even more insidious because everyone accepts it as normal. It is virtually impossible to stay lean and hard dining on American convenience food. The most commonly available foods at food courts, malls, highway rest stops, sporting events, drive-ins, college dormitories, cafeterias, take-out menus, business luncheons, office snack machines, buffets, weddings, bar mitzvahs, restaurants and delis is, in a word, hell. You cannot lose weight on it. You cannot be at your best on it. In one way or another it will eventually make you sick, tired, depressed or allergic, and it will, at the very least, most definitely make you fat.

One of the biggest success stories of recent years was Starbucks. Millions of Americans now start their day with 320 calories' (or more) worth of sugar and caffeine in some cutely named overpriced drink usually accompanied by any one of a cornucopia of pastries or Krispy Kreme doughnuts. (I know, I know, it's not *you* . . . but *someone* is buying that stuff.) Per capita sugar consumption in America is hovering around 145 pounds a year and rising, and other industrial nations aren't far behind. Get any bunch of friends together anywhere in America and suggest a friendly meal, and you're as likely as not to wind up with one of the top six:

• Pizza
• Fried chicken
• Hamburgers
• Hot dogs
• Chinese take-out
• Mexican

As often as not that'll be accompanied by potatoes fried in day-old rancid oil and a super-sized shake or soda that you could land a small seaplane in. A reporter for the *New York Post* recently accompanied teen idol Christina Aguilera on a photo shoot for *Seventeen* magazine, and reported that in one nine hour period she consumed the following: Chicken McNuggets, two large orders of fries from McDonald's, a chocolate shake, two slices of pizza, a Starbucks café mocha and a taco salad from Wendy's. And while Christina might be unusually gifted in the vocal department, she's not all that atypical in the eating department. (And, please, don't tell me how thin she is. She's also, as of this writing, nineteen years old. Talk to me again in twenty years.)

And it's not just kids. A recent study in *Obesity Research* explored the relationship between eating out and being fat. The researcher found that people who ate restaurant food more often consumed more calories and less fiber than those who ate out less often. Even when they controlled for potential confounding variables like physical activity, alcohol intake, socioeconomic level and smoking, the relationship held up. Restaurant food makes people fat, especially if it's the kind of restaurant food most people eat: fried chicken, burgers, pizza, Chinese, Mexican, and even non–fast food. And Americans are eating more of this stuff than ever before.

What's the likelihood that, living in this food environment, you can lose weight without effort? It would be like taking a recovering alcoholic and putting him in a bar twenty-four hours a day and expecting him to stay sober by accident. He could do it—and so can you—but not without a heightened consciousness of the real, tangible risks, and not without a serious strategy for how to deal with them.

So, if nothing seems to be working, go back to the drawing board. Take out that journal. Eliminate some food (dairy? grains?) for a trial period. And, for a while, count your calories. This *may* be just what the doctor ordered. It can be very empowering to know exactly what's going on, to face it down, understand it, tell the truth about it, shine that light on it and clean it up. If it remains unconscious, if you remain in the dark about it, it has power over you. You cannot deal with it effectively if you don't know what it is.

Now, does this kind of attention to detail mean you're going to have to actually be on a "diet," which is what Susan was resisting so strongly? I don't think that's the best way to look at it. Here's a better way: you now have the opportunity to shine a light on something that's been driving you nuts in order to understand it better, and out of that understanding is going to come power to change the very thing that's been making you crazy. You're going to develop a tool that's more valuable than any diet book, or any exercise program, and that tool is an understanding of what works for *your* body. And once you eliminate the silly idea that it has to be "fair," there's absolutely no stopping you.

Will you have to pay such close attention forever to what you're doing? Probably not. But you are going to have to work a bit to learn this new skill, and if you want to *master* it, you're going to have to *practice* it. Regularly. Till it becomes a habit. Rather than call that "dieting," I'd prefer to think of it as "skill acquisition."

Every year I go on vacation to St. Martin, and I take daily tennis lessons with Oliver Becaud, one of the great tennis pros in the world. And at the end of a week, I play much better than I did when I started. I'm actually almost "good." Then I go back to New York City, and don't play again until I return to St. Martin. And what do you think happens to those newly learned skills of mine?

You guessed it.

Suppose I invited *you* to a course in the Bahamas called "Eight Weeks to Perfect Tennis." Here's what you get to do: You come to tennis camp, you identify the problems in your serve, you work painstakingly on your backhand, you work on your groundstroke, you practice keeping your eye on the ball, you learn to anticipate where your opponent is going to hit and you generally put your game under a microscope for eight weeks.

Now, what happens to your game if, like me, you don't continue to practice once you get home? Would you expect to continue to be as good in six months as you were when you finished the course?

Any eight-week program—whether in tennis or dieting—is only as good as the habits it teaches you. If you don't continue to practice those habits, they atrophy. I think it's counterproductive to think of the kind of meticulous record keeping that I suggested Susan do for a few weeks as "dieting." I think it's far more productive and empowering to think of it like tennis camp. You're learning skills. But you need to continue to practice those skills once the eight weeks are over, or you will forget how to use them.

In this case, the main skill is amassing information on the way food affects you. Your weight, your mood, your energy. It's learning the *amounts* you need and the *kinds* you need. It's learning how to cut what you *don't* need from your "budget" and learning to choose the kind of fuels that are right for *your* engine and that further *your* goals. I want you to think of a "diet" as nothing more than a course in skill acquisition.

Right now, today, I want you to decide that you're going to stop flailing at the ball, hitting it every which way you can, running around without direction and just hoping it goes over the net. I want you to approach your weight loss and fitness scientifically, meticulously and fearlessly. I want you to forget about concepts like "fair" and "fate," and I want you to smile, laugh and realize that you can win this game, but to do so you need to know the rules, and the rules are different for each person. Sorry it's not fair, but really, so what? Who cares? We're going to level the playing field by arming you with information about the one person that matters in this endeavor, the one and only starring character in this play, the only person whose metabolism makes a difference here.

And that one person is you.

Ruining Your Metabolism?

The idea that people can "ruin" their metabolisms is a very disempowering notion. You can't ruin your metabolism. You *may* have some metabolic issues, and certainly understanding how your personal metabolism works can only help you in your weight loss journey, but this is very different from saying you "ruined" it.

For the sake of example, let's say you lose fifty pounds on a diet. Let's further assume that about half of that weight you lost is fat and half of it is muscle. (These percentages aren't exactly right, but they're good for the purpose of illustration.) You've now lost about twenty-five pounds of muscle and twenty-five pounds of fat. Now let's say that over time, you regain that same weight. Almost *all* of the regained weight is going to be fat, and virtually *none* of it is going to be muscle. So at the end of the day, you weigh the same as before, but your body composition is significantly different. You now have a significantly higher percentage of body fat.

Why does this matter? Simple. Most of your calories are "burned" by muscle tissue. Fat is basically metabolic dead weight. When you lose a lot of muscle, you lose one of your biggest allies in the war against fat. This shift in body composition is one of the things people refer to when they talk about their metabolism being "ruined" by dieting. To bring your metabolic rate up, one of the best things you can do is regain some of that lost muscle by adding weight training to your routine.

The other thing that frequently happens with constant yo-yo dieting is that you train your fat storage enzymes to be more efficient. When you starve yourself, those fat storage enzymes simply become more efficient at their job, an evolutionary strategy that protects you from dying during periods of famine. By exercising consistently and not eating more calories than you are using up—and, equally important, by eating the right *kind* of calories—you can retrain the fat-releasing enzymes to come out of hiding.

Most people in your situation have been trying to lose weight using a low-fat diet which is also low in protein and fiber. Unfortunately, that's probably exactly what you should *not* be eating. Low-fat diets are also high-carb diets, and a high-carb diet virtually guarantees that your body will be constantly producing high levels of insulin, also known as "the storage hormone." The body does not burn fat in the presence of high levels of insulin. What's more, yo-yo dieters, overweight people and sedentary people are much more likely to be insulin insensitive, meaning their bodies don't use insulin very well and require more than usual to do the job, virtually guaranteeing difficulty in losing fat. The solution? A moderate calorie diet with more protein, tons of vegetables, good fats like olive oil and fish and nuts, and far fewer carbohydrates than the usual low-fat diet.

The point is that there are specific positive actions you can take right now to work with almost any metabolic issue you may have as a result of your dieting history. Put these strategies into action right now, and maybe the next time you lose those fifty pounds it will be the last time you have to do it.

Dangerous Eating Situations

1. My Partner Overeats

OK, so you've finally got this eating thing down. More or less. You've spent a lot of hard time in the "diet wars," and you're a veteran. You've learned what foods make you feel good, which ones derail your weight loss efforts, which ones make you sleepy, and which ones give you energy. You've even got the sweet tooth thing down, at least most of the time (OK, maybe not 100 percent, but hey, it's a far cry from where you were a few weeks ago). In fact, you're feeling pretty good about things; you've even noticed the scale beginning to move. Your clothes are fitting better, and exercise is finally starting to feel like a habitual part of your life. Energy is up, and all told, you're feeling pretty darn good about things.

As well you should.

And then . . .

There's the Significant Other plunked down in front of the TV with beer, potato chips and pretzels.

Or . . .

You go out to dinner, and she can't resist the third piece of Italian bread. (And that's just for openers.)

Or . . .

You're at a wedding and that dessert buffet just keeps singing its siren song. Except you stay in your seat while he or she sings three-part harmony with it.

What do you do?

Think about it for a second, and then I'll tell you what I *think* you should do. But first, visualize the situation—there's no one reading this who hasn't experienced some version of it. Maybe it's not your significant other, maybe it's your kid, or your best friend at work. You can substitute whomever you want, but you know that sinking feeling I'm talking about when the person you care about is sitting across from you performing culinary suicide. OK, did you formulate your answer? Good. Here's mine:

You do . . .

Nothing.

And I'll tell you why.

But first you have to ask yourself the following question: What is the purpose of any intervention you might make?

Most people respond to that by saying they want to help their loved ones eat better. They want to impart their newfound information about health and feeling good and share that with the people around them. OK, great. That's a noble and worthwhile goal, and I'll tell you how to best achieve it. Some people would probably confess to the fact that watching others binge on stuff that they themselves only recently gave up triggers feelings of longing or craving that make it much harder for them to stay on track. That's an honest response, and probably a big part of what makes us crazy when our loved ones go off the deep end.

So why then do I say "Do nothing"?

For several reasons. One, did lecturing and preaching ever accomplish anything? Did it ever stop *you* from doing something that wasn't good for you? (Hint: Think "teenager.") Does it ever really work? More likely, it's just plain annoying.

Two, if your intention is truly to help your partner/friend/loved one, there are better ways to do it than nagging. Like by example. Take this to the bank: No one likes the food police. And you know what? No one likes *being* the food police. As a nutritionist and health coach, every time I go to some social event, I can count on at least some people looking up from their plates with guilty expressions and saying some version of, "I shouldn't be eating this, right?" It's not fun for them, and it's definitely not fun for me. So I'm giving you permission: Turn in your badge. There are better ways to accomplish what you're after.

Finally, if the thing that pushes your buttons is the fact that they can do it and you can't, well then . . . welcome to the world. It's a feeling every recovered alcoholic deals with every day of his or her life. Some people can eat this stuff, and some can't. You can't. Period. Deal with it.

There's a brilliant movie that no one ever heard of called *Resurrection*, based on a true story of a woman who finds that she has healing powers. She goes around the country at revival meetings, becomes a "laying-on of hands" preacher, and basically turns into a fairly obnoxious person who everyone winds up hating. In the end, she discovers that her gifts are best given to others subtly, without calling attention to them. She goes to a small town where no one ever heard of her and performs her miracles quietly and anonymously, simple acts of kindness and grace, without fanfare or pomp. It's a touching story, and one we would all do well to learn from.

Eat the way you need to eat for your own well-being. Get to be friends with that, get to own it as a method that works for *you*. Let your resulting good health and vitality be its own advertisement. You don't have to change the world, and you don't have to reform everyone else. You're not responsible for them, and they're not responsible for you. (You are, however, responsible for your own *feelings* about what they do.) Lead by example. Be someone the people around you admire and want to emulate.

Trust that they will come to you when and if they're ready. They will.

2. Eating With Family

Location, location, location.

If ever there was an activity to which the famous three-word mantra applied, it's dieting. It's hard to come up with another undertaking—with the possible exception of a summer house rental—that can be so easily wrecked by being in the wrong place with the wrong people. In this case the family dinner table.

With you as the centerpiece.

Eating with family comes in a cornucopia of flavors. There's the "home-for-the-holidays-dinner" flavor. There's the "going-out-with-the-in-laws" flavor. There's the "I-have-to-cook-for-six-people-and-they-think-this-healthy-stuff-tastes-like-rabbit-food" flavor. If you're thinking this doesn't sound like as much fun as Baskin-Robbins, you're on to something.

And each flavor comes with its own customized set of anxieties and pit-falls, especially made for you.

For some people, eating with family means something you do once or twice a year at holidays. For others, it's a nightly event. For some people it involves children. For others it involves in-laws. Some people feel very supported in their weight loss efforts by their families; others feel they are in the presence of a hostile, judging tribunal. In fact, one of the most dif-ficult areas for many people when they begin the Shape Up program is taking a hard and honest look at the support (or lack of support) coming from their immediate (and extended) family.

Since eating with family can mean so many things, it's hard to come up with one surefire strategy that will work for everyone in all situations. There is, however, one strategy you can use that will invariably make a dif-ference no matter what the particulars of the situation. And it can be summed up in one word:

Rehearsal.

Most of us know what we're going up against in situations where we've previously encountered trouble. For some it's the sight of the Thanksgiving table and relatives you haven't seen all year. For others it's a wedding buffet. For still others, it's the nightly specter of children com-plaining about the vegetables and a husband wanting to know why you're not eating the macaroni and cheese. Rehearsing a problem situation in your mind before it happens helps you to arm yourself with strategies, visualize yourself doing them and experience the positive results. That way you're not caught unprepared, and you can actually practice reacting to a variety of dangerous situations.

That's what coaches do with their athletes; it's what boxing trainers do with their fighters. "When he throws that left hook, you step in under and throw a right to the body." Studies have shown improvement in sports performance just by doing visualization exercises, for example, basketball players mentally practicing shooting baskets under various conditions. You can do the same thing with the family dinner table.

Of course to do this effectively, you have to be clear on what you want to happen. That's why I like using a tool I call the "proactive food journal." You can use this tool in your Shape Up journal any time you like. Pick a day, visualize what it's going to be like, where you're going to be and with whom. Think about what food is likely to be available. When you're likely to be hungry. What the circumstances are going to be. (Is your Aunt Tina going to be there insisting you try her special key lime pie? Are you going to be in a restaurant known for its crème brûlée and homemade breads? Are you going to be in a fast food restaurant taking care of six kids? Is your sister that you hate going to be there watching everything you eat and sitting in silent judgment?)

Now write down what you're going to eat. Decide in advance, and decide early in the day, or the night before. Visualize the situation. If there's temptation or anxiety, close your eyes and picture it. Hear in your mind's ear what people will say. See yourself responding in a way that would make you proud of yourself, whatever that is. It might mean allowing yourself one or two bites of something off your diet, it might mean being spartan. The point here is not *what* you choose, but *that* you choose it.

And that you then stick to it.

As Sondheim wrote, "The choice may have been mistaken. The choosing was not." The point here is to put you in charge of what happens, not the circumstances.

If you can accomplish that, you have begun a journey that not only will help you manage your weight but will empower you in all areas of your life.

Let the games begin.

3. Eating in Transit

In today's fast-paced and highly mobile world, few folks have the luxury of eating all their meals at an actual table. If they get one meal a day in at home it's a lot. In New York, where I live, street food stands do a brisk business and fast food and take-out shops are as common as monosyllables in an Adam Sandler flick. It's not uncommon to see people rushing through the streets, chomping furiously on anything they can hold in one hand, signaling for a taxi with the other.

It's not all that much different in cities less frenetic than New York. There are kids to chauffeur around, schedules to meet, meetings to go to, games to cheer at, ballet class, the gym, board meetings that last all afternoon, committees to chair and families to spend time with. The days of the Nortons and the Kramdens dropping in for coffee to break up the morning monotony are long over. What morning monotony? For better or worse, we live a Tasmanian devil of an existence that's exciting, maddening and frustrating all at the same time and, for those trying to eat well, a veritable minefield of potential disaster.

To make matters as bad as they could be, there seems to be an unwritten law which I call "the law of inverse quality." It states that the *quality of food goes down as portability and accessibility go up*. In other words, there ain't no organic fruits and vegetables at the food court, folks. Time and again my clients tell me that they are victimized by the sheer ubiquitousness of crummy, sugar-laden "pick-me-up" treats, processed meat sandwiches, stagnant salad bars, office snack machines, bad deli food, coffee and doughnut stands, fast food take-out, hot dogs, burgers, pretzels, bagels and other standard "take-me-with-you-as-you-travel" food.

And don't get me started on airplane food.

So what to do? Unless you've got access to a time machine, eating on the run, or at least on the move, is likely to remain a fact of life. The opportunity here is to become master of the circumstances rather than victimized by them. Like the great martial artists who learn to make lethal weapons out of such found objects as a paper clip or pencil, we need to learn to create healthy, nurturing meals out of commonly available "porta-foods." This food needs to be stuff that travels well, is available everywhere and still passes nutritional muster.

Here are my top-ten tips for how to do just that:

1. Think proactive.   Most of the trouble comes from waiting till you're in the middle of an emergency hunger situation before taking action (like being without food all afternoon and coming face to face with a convenient snack machine). A little planning goes a long way. If you know you're gonna be stuck in a meeting, take along something you can eat quickly and discreetly that will keep your blood sugar from plummeting and your cravings at bay.[1]

2. Lettuce is a great container. You can wrap some leftover chicken in a lettuce leaf and eat it in the car or anywhere else a sandwich would work. Throw on some tomatoes and a drizzle of olive oil and you've got a decent mini-meal. A couple of leaves of red-leaf lettuce make a great wrap and the contents are limited only by your imagination.

3. Find healthy food that travels well. Some suggestions: cottage cheese, yogurt, celery, peppers, carrots, and apples. Throw some berries into a Tupperware with some cottage cheese and nuts and take it in the car with you. In a pinch, the high-protein, low-carb snack bars beat the pants off of standard snack machine food.

4. Make it the night before. (This is the corollary of "think proactively"). At my house, we sometimes bake a week's worth of sweet potatoes on a Sunday and take them with us as snacks during the week. They're as portable as you can get, they taste great cold and they are a veritable vitamin store.

5. Think unusual foods. Sally Fallon, the great exponent of traditional nourishing foods, says that the best "energy bar" is a homemade, nitrous-free, lean-meat sausage. If you can find a local butcher who still makes sausage like this, grab it.

6. Think outside the box. One person's unusual is another person's delicious. Experiment. I've found that cutting up an apple and eating it with a single serving of tuna adds crunchiness and sweetness to the tuna that makes it a taste treat. Ditto with celery. A single serving can of tuna can be bought almost anywhere and also goes great with that baked sweet potato you made last Sunday. Or discover your own combinations. You can always find nuts, cheese, fruit and seeds. Use them creatively, or eat them right out of the package. Hint: String cheese is a really easy snack to take on the run and is available everywhere.

7. Use your blender. Many office-bound people forget that a blender is an easy accessory to keep in a desk or in the company kitchen. In a pinch, packaged meal replacements like Met-Rx, Myoplex, and Lee Labrada's Lean Body can be made quickly and are way better for you than most of the stuff at the food court.[2]

8. Ditto for the microwave. It only takes about four minutes to make real oatmeal (not the packaged kind), and you can add some berries or soy milk and take it with you anywhere in a plain take-out coffee cup. Plus, if you sweeten it a little with a good maple syrup and then let it get cold, it almost tastes like dessert.

9. Make a list.   Until you get good at this, don't try to think on your feet. Make a list in advance of possible combinations that might be available while you're traveling or that you could easily take with you. One of my favorites is celery with cream cheese. There's got to be at least half a dozen others just as good. Discover them.

10. Vegetable juice is a lifesaver.   When all else fails, have a V-8. Fresh vegetable juice is always better, and possibly one of the best things you can put in your body, but in a pinch there's always canned tomato juice and V-8. It takes the edge off your appetite and quenches cravings like nothing else around, and you can get it anywhere. Add celery, leave out the vodka, and you'll almost feel like it's happy hour.

4. Dating and Dieting

Few experiences seem so fraught with danger for my female friends as the prospect of mixing the early phase of a dating relationship with an ongoing weight management program. It's no picnic for men either.

While men seem to have only one simple rule to worry about—"Don't order the spaghetti on a first date"—women, as usual, seem to have a far more complex situation on their proverbial plate.

On the one hand there's the issue of how to maintain a weight loss program while going out socially without appearing to be picky, hard-to-please or, worse yet, on the road to an eating disorder. On the other hand, there's the issue of how to enjoy food with gusto without appearing to be someone who doesn't care about their appearance.

And how do you strike the proper balance between being able to have a good time and do fun things in a social atmosphere and still being true to a commitment to either shrink or maintain a waistline that doesn't seem to want to overlook your bad behavior at the buffet?

What to do, what to do . . .

This is a time when all that spiritual, new-agey advice about "just being yourself" is about as welcome as Monica Lewinsky at a Hillary Clinton fundraiser. You want answers, and you want solutions, and you want them now. Before the doorbell rings.

In dating and dieting, like so many other areas of life, a little preparation and planning go a long way towards making life easier.

First of all, remember the 80/20 rule (sometimes known as the 90/10 rule, depending on how strict your superego is). It goes like this: What you do 80 (or 90) percent of the time is what makes the difference in the long run. Translated to weight loss, it means that going out for a special Sunday brunch date that involves pancakes and bagels is probably not going to undo everything you've worked for if you've worked for it consistently most of the time. If the brunch detour is taken only 10 percent of the time, it might knock a few apples off the apple cart, but it won't turn the whole cart upside down.

Second, don't starve yourself in anticipation of the big dinner date during which you're sure you're going to overeat. Arriving hungry is a definite recipe for disaster. Here's why: Skipping meals or undereating during the day is perceived by the body as starvation, and it primes the fat storage enzymes for an emergency situation. Since you arrive at dinner starving, you're far more likely to overeat, which in turn triggers both high levels of insulin release and lots of activity on the part of the enzymes that store fat. A much better strategy is to eat small, sensible meals during the day and arrive at the dinner date just hungry enough to be able to eat, but not starving enough to eat the bread basket.

Third, you can minimize the damage in a recreational meal by doing a few easy things. Eat the whole meal—from the proverbial soup to nuts—within one hour of starting. This technique, pioneered by Drs. Richard F. and Rachael F. Heller in their "Carbohydrate Addict's" program, helps keep insulin levels from going out of control. The Hellers also recommend beginning the meal with a salad and dividing the rest of the meal into equal parts protein, fiber (vegetables) and starchy or sugary carbohydrates (potatoes, rice, or dessert). I'd add to that the recommendations to include some good fat like olive oil or nuts and to keep the starch part as low as you can. The point, however, is to keep the total glycemic load of the meal relatively low. The inclusion of the protein, fat and fiber helps keep the overall effect on blood sugar and insulin levels in the reasonable range. And for best effect, eat the carbs last.

Teachers are familiar with a concept called "overlearning." It means, briefly, that if you know a subject cold before the midterm, you're more likely to do well on it, even allowing for the fact that stress may make you temporarily forget stuff you'd easily recall under less tense conditions. Dating can be a big source of anxiety, and most of us—men and women—find that when stressed we are *least* likely to do what's difficult and *most* likely to revert to what's comfortable and easy. That's why building the kind of eating habits and style that support you in your goals is so important to do. The more those habits are second nature to you, the more likely you'll be able to incorporate them even when you're worried about something (or someone) else.

And when all else fails, as an internal pep talk, remember this: However much you *think* he's paying attention to what you're eating, he's probably not. In fact, if in between bites you just keep asking the right questions and nodding your head at the answers, he'll be far too busy thinking about what a wonderful conversationalist you are to worry about anything else. (Men: Same goes for you.)

When Is Food More Than Food?
Emotional Eating 101

OK, let's face it. When you were a little baby, and things didn't go well, and you needed comfort and love, your mother didn't bring you a plate of asparagus.

From before you can remember, deep in the DNA of your unconsciousness, food has always been conditioned to some amalgamation of love, security, safety and/or comfort.

It begins with milk—the real kind, not the fake kind you get in the supermarket. It had more fat than the bottled kind, less protein and was warm and sweet and soothing to your infant taste buds—in short, it was exactly what your body needed, and it washed away the pain of hunger. Plus, since it didn't just materialize from the sky, its delivery usually meant that someone who cared about you was around to provide it. A nice double whammy in the conditioning department.

Bingo. Home run. An association embedded in your cortex, a Pavlovian field demonstration, and an equation is forever formed: Food equals love.

And, boy, did you learn that lesson well.

And in one fashion or another, it's probably always been this way. No matter how much we evolved over the past few million years, one truth remains: The human infant has one of the longest periods of helplessness of any mammal. Without a caretaker, it won't survive. This serves a double evolutionary purpose—not only does it bond the infant to the mother, but it bonds the caretaker to the cared for. It is the building block molecule of the social contract, and without it, bad stuff happens.

Fast-forward twenty to eighty years from the cradle. You feel pain. You feel loneliness. You feel frustration. You feel empty. What do you reach for?

I'll give you a hint. It's not broccoli.

Food and love have been celebrated and ritualized in one way or another for as long as there has been community. Holiday meals. Wedding banquets. Dinner dates. Family gatherings. "*Eat*, darling!" Birthday parties.

Tribal hunts and subsequent feasts. Celebration of the Mass. Passover. Ramadan. You name it, if there is social meaning to it, there's going to be food involved. Food is so powerfully conditioned to feelings that it seems like an impossibility to consider food apart from its context. For many people, the mere thought of a favorite food evokes powerful associations fusing image, taste, sensation, feeling, emotion, and memory into a textured nugget of experience that is near impossible to separate into its constituent parts.

Indeed, this is precisely the mosh pit into which most folks attempting to change their eating habits fall, and from which many never successfully climb out.

In other words, when the boyfriend dumps you, buttered stringbeans and grilled fish just don't cut it.

Oh that it did. Oh that comfort and console, soothe and calm could be found at the end of a forkful of vegetables rather than crème brûlée. Would that at the end of a day full of stress and anxiety, that pint of gourmet ice cream in the freezer did not sing its siren song quite so loudly. Would that the voices in our heads chanting the familiar litany ("It's not going to kill me," "I deserve it after what I've been through today," "I can start tomorrow") were not so well miked.

But they are. And if you're going to be successful in managing your weight, you need to stop waiting for them to shut up and learn how to live amidst their annoying chatter.

One of the most valuable lessons I ever learned happened when I stopped smoking. Like many people, I figured eventually the craving would stop, I wouldn't think about cigarettes so much and the habit would just sort of go away by itself. Big mistake. It's been over fifteen years and even now (very rarely, it's true, but occasionally), I'll get an urge to fill my lungs with irritating, carcinogenic, cancer-producing cigarette smoke. Don't ask me why. Who cares? The important thing is that I don't do it. What I learned was that if you wait for the little voices saying "taste me, taste me" or "smoke me, smoke me" to shut up, you're in for a really long wait, and you will probably never stop doing what you want to stop doing. The real action, I found, is not in trying to make the voices go away. It's in learning how to disempower them, or at least live with them in peaceful cohabitation. The voices can go on—in fact, they *will* go on, whether you want them to or not—but you don't have to give them the power to run your life. What I learned when I finally stopped smoking fifteen years ago was that I could *have* the impulse to do something stupid and destructive like smoke a cigarette, and yet not empower it. I could notice it, watch it, experience it, and let it float by rather than being sucked into the vacuum of its pull.

That's empowerment.

And it doesn't necessarily come cheap.

From infancy, we cry when we're hungry and stop when we're fed. We learn that the pain and discomfort of hunger can be stopped by a bottle, and replaced with the warm, fuzzy comfort of a full tummy, often accompanied by affection and a soothing voice. Food becomes conditioned to the easing of pain and discomfort, becomes the means by which we soothe emotional distress, becomes the tool with which we self-medicate our anxieties and hurts and desperations and loneliness, becomes the surrogate for human contact or the bridge with which we form connections. Food is celebration: Thanksgiving, Christmas, birthdays, holidays. Food is solace. Food is social: gatherings, lunches, buffets, dinners, dating. Food is familiar. Food is solitary.

Food becomes a friend who is reliably, consistently, dependably always there.

No wonder dieters feel they are going mad.

What's more, like a drug, the most destructive foods feed addictions. High-carbohydrate, high-sugar convenience and comfort foods produce not only corresponding high blood sugar and insulin levels, leading to even more cravings, but higher levels of serotonin. In other words, "instant Prozac." In sensitive people, particularly those who may have low serotonin levels to begin with, a carbohydrate binge is the equivalent of self-medicating. I've heard more than a few folks describe the feeling after a sugar binge as being almost "high."

So what to do?

First let's frame the question.

Is there warmth and comfort without food? Sometimes.

But more important, is there warmth and comfort without self-destruction?

Here are the top ten things I've learned to ask when it seems like nothing else will do the trick but the food you want the most and need the least.

- What am I really feeling?
- Can I just *be* with this feeling?
- If I eat this food or go on this binge, what is it costing me?
- What's really important to me right now?
- Is there a better way to take care of myself?
- What gift can I give myself right now that won't cost me my power?
- How can I nurture myself right now without hurting myself?
- If I were a child right now, how would I like to be comforted?

• What could I do right now that would make me feel good tomorrow?

And finally, and perhaps most important of all . . .

• If I *do* eat this comfort food, can I savor it, enjoy it, relish it, and then let it go . . . without beating myself up and without giving up on my commitment?

If the answer to the last one is yes, well then . . .
Bon appétit.

A Nutritional Cure for PMS?

Up to 150 different symptoms have been linked with PMS. They can range from barely noticeable to downright debilitating. And to this day, though PMS has been a well-researched entity since at least the 1980s (if not before), many physicians still believe that it doesn't really exist and that it is "all in your mind."

Well, it's not.

During the time before your period, there are powerful hormonal upsets that influence mood, craving, and water retention and, for some sensitive people, create maddeningly difficult emotional personality changes. There is no single cause that explains PMS in every case. PMS seems to have at least four "types." Obviously each of these types is shorthand for a constellation of symptoms, but here's an easy way to remember them: A for anxiety, B for bloating (sometimes called H for hydration), C for cramps, and D for depression. Some folks like to add the all-too-familiar fifth type, E (for everything).

That there is a nutritional link to PMS seems almost inarguable. Researchers have shown that the typical PMS sufferer consumes 275 percent more sugar, 62 percent more refined carbohydrates, 78 percent more sodium, 79 percent more dairy products, 52 percent less zinc, 77 percent less magnesium, and 53 percent less iron than non–PMS sufferers.

One theory that's been put forth to explain at least some of the familiar constellation of symptoms is the theory of "estrogen dominance." Basically it says this: When the ideal ratio of estrogen to progesterone is thrown way out of whack, things go south fast. Nearly all of the common PMS symptoms, such as bloating, weight gain, headaches and backache, are also symptoms of a relative excess of estrogen. Is there a dietary connection here as well? You betcha. Many foods that naturally contain estrogen—like meat and dairy products—are frequently from animals which are loaded with synthetic hormones, providing a nice double whammy; add to that the hundreds of "environmental estrogens"—chemicals found in our environment, food and water supply—that mimic estrogen in the body, and you begin to get an idea of our chronic level of exposure.

It gets worse. Estrogens can suppress the action of dopamine, an important neurotransmitter involved in creating relaxation and alertness. Dopamine also helps prevent sodium and water retention, so if it's suppressed, guess what happens. And some research has found that the serotonin levels of women with PMS were significantly lower than those without, which might account for some common symptoms like depression and anxiety. Stress, a constant fact of life for many women, can make matters worse by affecting hormone production and further upsetting the balance. Caffeine amplifies the effects of stress and contributes to anxiety, tension and irritability. Women who consume large amounts of coffee are far more likely to suffer from PMS. Low thyroid function might be a factor as well. A study in the *New England Journal of Medicine* showed that 51 of 54 PMS sufferers showed low thyroid status compared to zero out of 12 for a control group.

Is there a nutritional cure for this complex hormonal-neurotransmitter stew? Well, I don't know that I'd go as far as to say "cure," but there certainly are some strategies that are well worth trying and have provided relief for an awful lot of women who have been willing to experiment with them. Following are some of the best.

1. **Cut out sugar.** Symptom-free women consume far less refined sugar and refined carbohydrates (and dairy products) than those with symptoms.
2. **Cut out coffee.** Among other things, caffeine suppresses the neurotransmitter adenosine, which in turn calms nerve receptors. Without adenosine, nerve receptors can become overly reactive, leading to irritability, mood swings and a worsening of symptoms.
3. **Exercise.** It promotes both circulation and the removal of toxins from the body, plus it raises the level of endorphins, which have a relaxing and mood-improving effect.
4. **Reduce stress.** Do whatever it takes, but take this mandate seriously. Part of that is getting enough sleep. No kidding.

5. **Take the PMS cocktail:** 1,000 mg of evening primrose oil, 400 mg of magnesium, and 100 mg of B-6, taken twice a day, beginning about five to ten days before your period. Though less than optimal intakes of many nutrients may make symptoms worse, nearly everyone agrees that these three are critical.

6. **Consider chasteberry.** Also known as vitex, this is the number one herb used throughout Europe to help relieve symptoms of PMS. It acts directly on the pituitary gland to stimulate the secretion of leutinizing hormone, which in turn stimulates the secretion of progesterone, helping to create a more hormonally balanced state. And it can be used along with the supplements mentioned.

7. **Try calcium.** Some studies have shown that calcium supplementation may help with PMS symptoms (about 1,000 mg daily). Supplements may be better than dairy, for reasons mentioned above.

8. **Reduce alcohol.** Seriously.

9. **Get some sun.** Lack of sunlight (or full-spectrum light) seriously reduces serotonin levels, contributing to depression and lack of energy.

Above all, be good to yourself, experiment with these strategies and give them enough time to work. It'll be worth the effort.

Inner Voices, Inner Chatter

Is Your Inner Voice Holding You Back?

A client recently came to me—let's call him Pete—who weighed in the mid-200s. Heavy most of his life, he was finally ready to do something to change his high-stress, eat-on-the-run, junk-food lifestyle and begin taking care of himself. Since I no longer take on personal training clients, I worked with him on his nutrition program and sent him to one of the best trainers I know in New York, Bill Humphries.

To make a long story short, after about six months this guy, who could barely walk a flight of steps without puffing when we first met, was running an eight-and-a-half-minute mile on the treadmill. He dropped forty pounds and looks and feels better than he ever has.

Now here's the thing.

Pete's dad was an ex-marine, and heavily valued traditionally masculine behavior—"toughing it out," "boys don't cry," Monday night football . . . you get the drift. Pete's a kind of an "artsy," creative type, who felt like he could never really please his dad in the "testosterone-driven-activity" department. What's more, Pete's early attempts at sports weren't very successful, and his father teased him mercilessly for his poor performance.

On more than one occasion, his father said to him, only half-jokingly, "Man, Pete . . . you run like a *girl!*"

That comment, in the way that certain childhood incidents have of sticking to the flypaper of our unconscious and remaining there long past the time that we bother to think about them, has stayed with Pete all of his life and, in some not fully understood way, has kept him well stocked in negative feelings about exercise for all of his adult life.

Not anymore.

As he recounted what I've just told you, he had tears in his eyes. "That 8.5-mile meant more to me than you could possibly know," he said.

That got me thinking.

Pete had an inner voice telling him that he looked silly when he exercised. That he'd never be any good at it, that he "ran like a girl." What his trainer, Bill Humphries, had done was not just teach him how to run, but somehow get him past something that had been holding him back and keeping him imprisoned in a body that he was finally ready to leave behind. (That, by the way, is great coaching in action.)

How many of us have similar incidents, similar self-evaluations, gathering cobwebs in our minds' closets, preventing us from really breaking through and having the bodies that we want to have? Or, for that matter, the relationships? Or the income? Or just plain keeping us from feeling good about the stuff we *do* have?

How many of us were called "fat" and believed it was a judgment about us for all time? How many believed—and still believe—that the number on the scale makes a major statement about who we are? How many are caught up in intricate entanglements of relationships that would be severely threatened if we were ever to break out of the role our weight assigns to us and become something different?

How many have people in our lives who would really be threatened if we began to shine?

Now this isn't to say that there aren't real influences on weight that all of us struggle with: genetics, hormones, dieting history, metabolism, physiology, cravings, neurotransmitter levels, you name it. But it's also worth checking out whether some of these stories we tell ourselves—the chatter of our inner voices—keep us imprisoned in the past or in an image of ourselves that no longer serves or nurtures us.

Here are my candidates for the top ten list of stories from the "inner voices" that just might be holding you back regarding weight:

1. I'll always be fat.
2. I'm not attractive.
3. No one will ever want me at this weight.
4. I have no self-control.
5. It's my family's (or husband's, son's, father's, mother's, lover's, boyfriend's, girlfriend's) fault.
6. I can't really be happy till I lose (xxxx) pounds.
7. I'm not athletic.
8. I deserve it; one slice is not kill me.
9. Fat people aren't sexy.
10. I'll start tomorrow.

Any of them sound familiar?

If so, maybe you and that chatterbox in your head ought to sit down and have a heart-to-heart.

Maybe it's time for him to move out.

After all, he's lived in there long enough.

Notes

1. Some celery sticks and a small jar of peanut butter for dipping. String cheese and an apple. Or, what is arguably the greatest, and cheapest, health food in the world, a can of sardines.

2. These are shakes that come in an envelope. Mix with water and you've got a very decent meal replacement. You can prepare them as is or customize them—adding berries, for example. The better ones beat the pants off those canned meal replacements, and they take up less room in your bag or briefcase.

WEIGHT LOSS AND THE PLEASURE PRINCIPLE

19

I had a psychology professor in graduate school who once demonstrated this principle to our class in a way that I'm sure none of us who were present will ever forget. He had all of the chairs in our classroom hooked up to an unseen device, which, when he pushed a button, would deliver a harmless but annoying little shock to the seat of the chairs. He asked the class to stand in front of their chairs and explained to us that he was going to do a demonstration which might cause us a bit of discomfort but was perfectly safe. Once everyone agreed, he asked the class to take their seats. We sat down and promptly felt this annoying, surprising little shock. We all jumped up immediately. He then smiled and said, "OK, you can sit down. I promise I won't do that again." We all looked around the room at each other a little hesitantly, but we all eventually sat down. At which point he shocked us *again*. After we all jumped up in disbelief, he said, "OK, OK, you can sit down now. *Really*, this time I mean it. Look, I'll even disable the shock button. You can sit down now and nothing will happen." Well, this time, no one sat down. Even when he showed us that he had disabled the button and walked away from the device, no one was willing to be the first to sit back down.

He had made his point memorably: People believe their *experience* before they believe their intellect. As that demonstration showed us, the *experience* of being shocked had far more impact on our behavior than the *intellectual idea* that we wouldn't be shocked anymore.

If this sounds like something you can relate to, then you already understand intuitively something about conditioning. Conditioning is what happens when a bell rings at dinnertime and after a while you salivate when you hear the bell. Conditioning is what happens when a ballplayer rubs a lucky charm before throwing a perfect game and then believes he has to have that charm in his pocket before he can pitch again. Conditioning is what happens when a song you heard a lot when you first fell in love continues to elicit a little fluttery response in your tummy, even when you hear it twenty years later. Conditioning is going on in your life every moment of every day. But the things that have the most effect on your behavior are the things that are most strongly and immediately associated not with concepts, but with pleasure or pain (like the electric shock you got when you plugged in the toaster).

Virtually everyone who is struggling with fat is also struggling with some very powerful conditioning, and understanding how the pleasure-pain principle works can be a big help in breaking through some of the barriers that may be holding you back unconsciously. Here's why: Living in a body you don't like is undoubtedly associated with a certain amount of pain. But it's "long distance" pain. And doing something to change the situation takes time. You don't get to see results right away. Sure, having a fitter, leaner body would be a great source of pleasure to you, but it's a long distance pleasure. It's not here *right now*, in this moment.

Contrast that to the experience of eating some comfort food. Satisfying a craving for chocolate is associated with pleasure. Ordering from the dessert tray is associated with pleasure. And it's *immediate* pleasure. You can have it *right now*, this instant. Saying no to that is associated with *immediate pain*. No matter that you may pay for that comfort food later, later is later and now is now. In the battle in your brain between an *immediate pleasure* and a *far-off reward* the immediate pleasure gets the edge every time. If it's a choice between whether to avoid the *immediate* pain of turning down that Krispy Kreme doughnut or to chip away at the more remote *conceptual* pain of being trapped in a body you don't like, guess what wins out? You grab that doughnut and worry about the long-term goals later.

So in order to start making choices that support the long distance goal of having a healthier, fitter, leaner body, you have to start using this conditioning process to your own advantage. That means finding a way to associate *pain* to the experience of eating junk and *pleasure* to the experience of pushing it away. You have to take an active part in your own conditioning.

For years, as part of my own personal fitness program, I jogged. I was never a great runner, but it was something I needed to do to keep my weight under control and to keep my cardiovascular health. And as a personal trainer I needed to "walk the walk" and live the example. So I made myself do it, even though I never particularly liked it.

Then, like most people, a point came when I just got lazy and stopped doing it for a while. It got harder and harder to go back to it. I'd make myself do it, or I'd get my personal trainer to make me do it, but it was more and more of a struggle. And since I was doing it less, I felt like when I *did* do it I had to do it more intensely just to make it "count." This led to harder (but less frequent) runs, which I hated even more. The experience of running, never a particularly pleasurable one, had now become strongly associated with pain. And I knew that as long as this was the case, my running days were numbered.

So here's what I did.

I thought about what I really like to do, which is to relax, think and listen to music. Those are pretty pleasurable experiences for me. So I went down to the gym in my building, got on the treadmill and set the speed for a very easy walk—for me, that was four miles per hour. I put on my headset, and listened to tapes and let my mind drift, writing chapters of this book in my head, listening to music or lectures, preparing my radio show or just spacing out. And I walked for forty-five minutes. Not once did I increase the speed. By the end of the forty-five minutes I felt great. Refreshed and rejuvenated and not at all exhausted. The next day I did the same thing. I started finding special tapes that I hadn't had a chance to listen to before and I made a deal with myself that I'd only listen to them while walking on the treadmill. If I found tapes that I really wanted to hear, I would actually begin to look forward to my time on the treadmill, since this was the only time I'd get to listen to stuff I really liked listening to. I did this for a month or so. The treadmill experience was now becoming associated with pleasure. Eventually I began to inject short interval runs of a tenth of a mile with the walking program. The intervals felt great. I never felt like I was pounding away, never felt like I was making myself do something I hated and actually got to where I was looking forward to the daily time on the treadmill. I had taken an experience—doing cardio—that had become associated with pain for me and had reconditioned it to be associated with pleasure.

As long as an activity like eating foods you know you shouldn't eat—or smoking cigarettes, or doing drugs—is more strongly associated in someone's life with the *avoidance of immediate pain* than it is with pleasure, it's going to be very hard to give up. What we need to do is start conditioning *pleasure* to the experience of, for example, walking away from a dessert tray and *pain* to the experience of eating junk. What we need to do is start associating *positive actions* that we take with *pleasure* while associating *negative actions* with *pain*.

Maybe you do that by creating a pleasurable experience for yourself as soon as you walk away from the table. Maybe the minute you turn down that plate of ice cream you take a warm, relaxing bath. Or maybe you get to sit with a book. Or listen to a favorite CD. You have to be creative here, because you're trying to literally condition yourself to have a pleasurable association to an action that in the past has been unpleasant, just as I did with my treadmill experience. The idea is to make saying no to junk a *positive* experience.

And no, that does not mean you will never be able to eat "recreationally" again, or that you will never be able to enjoy Sunday brunch or occasionally overindulge, or eat a big piece of birthday cake. (You might not *want* to do that a lot, but you can.) But it *does* mean that you need to break the automatic associations that have been building up for all these years between eating junk and feeling better and between saying no and pain.

Breaking these associations—and putting new ones in their place—can be one of the most powerful tools you can develop, and it will serve you amazingly well not only in building a better body but in other areas of life. Let me tell you how it worked for me when I stopped smoking. As any smoker knows, smoking is associated with immediate pleasure (but long-term pain). Saying no to a cigarette once you're hooked is, in the immediate present, a painful experience. The trick for the smoker who wants to become an *ex-smoker* is to begin to associate *unpleasantness* with *smoking* and *pleasure* with *not smoking*. But how do you do that?

Putting a "Chink in the Link"

Most overeating behaviors are actually *chains* or *links* of behaviors that we do automatically and unconsciously. Think: reaching for a cigarette when you're nervous, or staring vacantly at the open refrigerator while you mindlessly munch, or grabbing for some chocolate at the first sign of stress. One way to make a change is to put a *break* in that chain of automatic behaviors, forcing yourself to have to do something different somewhere along the well-traveled route. I call this inserting a *"chink in the link."* It breaks the "automatic-ness" of the chain and also throws a little consciousness into the mix. It's the beginning of reconditioning some of those powerful pain/pleasure associations.

In the stop smoking program I went to, here's how we put chinks in the link. First, we wrapped our cigarettes up in paper and put a rubber band around them. We were still allowed to smoke, but we had to unwrap the cigarettes first, unfold the paper and write on it the time of day and the circumstances (after breakfast? after coffee? after dinner? after sex?). Then we had to rate the importance of that cigarette on a scale of 1–10. Afterwards, we wrapped them back up again and put them away. The second week, another step was added: We still had to unwrap the cigarettes, unfold the paper, write on it the time of day, rate the importance of the cigarette on a scale of 1–10—*but then we had to wait exactly five minutes before smoking it.* The third week, same routine, but this time we had to *leave the room we were in and go somewhere else to have the cigarette,* preferably somewhere small and cramped, like a tiny bathroom, or somewhere distinctly uncomfortable, like a drafty hallway. In addition, we had to promise not to socialize, talk on the phone or read while having that cigarette. The cigarette really had to be a time-out; only after we stubbed it out could we return to whatever it was we were doing.

All during the program, we were instructed to make time to do the things we loved to do the most—whether renting movies, reading books, going boating, whatever; but *not* to smoke while doing them. We were still allowed to smoke, but we were breaking the association between cigarettes and these pleasant activities. As the program progressed, the situations in which we were *allowed* to have our cigarettes became progressively more unpleasant, while the situations in which we *could not* have our cigarettes became progressively more enjoyable. By the end of the six-week program, smoking didn't feel the same to most of us. The very fact of having to wrap, unwrap and rate the cigarettes had put a chink in the link of automatic behaviors. We had broken the back of the automatic associations that sustained the smoking habit and begun to put new ones in their place. The fact that most of us were beginning to be able to breathe for the first time in years and feeling more powerfully in control of our own fates only reinforced the new associations to non-smoking that we were slowly developing.

In the same way, you want to begin to associate pain to the experience of eating stuff you really don't need to be eating (that is, if you want to get to your goal). How do you do that? Well, maybe you take out a picture of yourself that really hurts you to look at, and you force yourself to look at it *while* you eat that junk food. Do that often enough, and believe me, eating the junk food will become associated with enough pain to make it easier to stop, especially if stopping simultaneously becomes associated with doing something pleasurable.

Another way to help this process along is to restructure the way you think about eating. Instead of telling yourself that you're denying yourself a food, how about telling yourself you're giving yourself a gift? That you're giving yourself the first in a series of gift certificates that, if saved up, will be redeemable for a body you'll be a lot more comfortable in and that you'll like a whole lot more.

Conditioning, as the great motivational coach Tony Robbins points out, is going to go on all the time whether you like it or not. So why not begin, right this moment, to take an active part in it? To help your brain make the associations that support and nourish you in the goals you want to achieve?

Before doing the Shape Up program, your life was a roller coaster. After doing the Shape Up program, guess what? It's *still* going to be a roller coaster.

Only this time, instead of lying passively on the tracks, you're gonna be riding in the front car.

A PLAN FOR LIFE

One of the most discouraging aspects of weight loss is the inevitable slips. Everyone has them. For some people, an occasional slip engenders an all-out binge, followed by guilt, self-recrimination, a sense of powerlessness and a feeling of "what's the use?"

Sound familiar?

I call it "falling off the diet wagon," and if you change how you think about it, you don't need to be victimized by it anymore.

To illustrate what I'm talking about, let's look at a simple children's board game called Chutes and Ladders. Here's how it works: You use a spinner to advance over 100 spaces on the board. Every so often, there are ladders, which leapfrog you over a lot of spaces, advancing you towards the winner's spot. However, equally prominent along the path are chutes, which send the player back in the opposite direction.

Some kids play this game with a laissez-faire, "whatever" attitude, taking life as it comes with all its ups and downs, pitfalls and triumphs. They learn the wonderful moral of the game, which is that half of the secret to life is just showing up: Keep playing the game, throwing the dice, and eventually you'll get where you're going.

Some, however, get very upset when they land on a chute. They're ready to quit the game, pick up their proverbial marbles and go home. For some reason, they believe that life isn't supposed to have any chutes, so when they land on them they are very disappointed and feel like giving up.

Weight loss is like a huge game of Chutes and Ladders.

In dealing with hundreds of clients over the years, I've discovered that the biggest difference between the winners and the losers in the weight loss wars isn't really whether or not people have slips and go off their program. (In fact, it's not really a question of "if" they have them, it's a question of "when," since just about everyone has them.)

What really makes the difference is how you deal with them when they happen.

Here's an example: You've been absolutely wonderful on your eating plan for three weeks, sticking to your exercise routine and feeling pretty terrific. You goes to your best friend's wedding and have a glass of wine. Before you know it, someone is insisting you try those delicious little canapés, and before the wedding singer can say "Tanta Elka Cuts the Cake," you've managed to down about 4,000 unwanted calories from stuff you wouldn't have been caught dead looking at during the past couple of weeks: pâtés, desserts, breads, stuffings, you name it.

Most people think that's where the action stops. Actually, it's where the real action begins.

First, a reality check. Have you done a lot of damage? Not really. Maybe you put on a pound or two. Big deal. You can knock it off in no time and go right back to work on yourself.

So what's the problem?

The problem isn't what you did, but what you make it mean. You tell yourself that your transgression means that you have no willpower, that you will never succeed, that your efforts are in vain.

In other words, you hit a chute and now you want to stop the game.

Let me suggest something more empowering.

Suppose, instead, you learn to see life's occasional chutes as just that, stumbling blocks that everyone hits on their personal path to personal power, nothing to be afraid of and certainly nothing to give a lot of "meaning" to.

So you hit a chute. Next roll of the dice, you might hit a ladder.

Most important of all, you can't win the game unless you keep on playing.

And every minute gives you a new chance for another try at the spinner.

Take it. And don't look back.

APPENDIX

Alternate Exercise Programs for Advanced Beginners, Intermediate and Advanced

Intermediate Exercise Routine: Home-Based—Dumbbells

Monday, Wednesday, Friday

Light warm-up: jogging in place or fast walk
Crunches
10-minute run

- Squats
- One-arm rows } Circuit 1
- Chest press

- Squats
- One-arm rows } Circuit 2
- Chest press

Three-minute jump rope, free dance, or two sets of 20–25 jumping jacks with a very short rest between sets

- Bicep curls
- Lateral raises } Circuit 3
- Tricep dips

- Bicep curls
- Lateral raises } Circuit 4
- Tricep dips

Three-minute jump rope, free dance, or two sets of 20–25 jumping jacks with a very short rest between sets

- Push-ups
- Squats } Circuit 5

- Push-ups
- Squats } Circuit 6

Ten-minute run with two-minute cooldown

Tuesday, Thursday

Forty-five-minute slow, comfortable jog

Saturday or Sunday (or both)

Something fun and active. Tennis? Golf? Hike? Tae-Bo? Yoga?

Intermediate Exercise Routine: Gym-Based

Monday, Wednesday, Friday

Light warm-up: Jogging in place or fast walk
Crunches
Ten-minute run on treadmill

- Cable rows (or Lat pull-downs)
- Incline press machine } Circuit 1

- Cable rows (or Lat pull-downs)
- Incline press machine } Circuit 2

Three-minute treadmill—push yourself

- Leg extensions
- Leg curls
} Circuit 3

- Leg extensions
- Leg curls
} Circuit 4

Three-minute treadmill—push yourself

- Bicep curls
- Shoulder press machine (or Lateral raises)
- Tricep press-downs
} Circuit 5

- Bicep curls
- Shoulder press machine (or Lateral raises)
- Tricep press-downs
} Circuit 6

Ten-minute run with the last two minutes cool-down
Stretch

Tuesday, Thursday

Forty-five-minute slow, comfortable jog

Saturday or Sunday (or both)

Something fun and active. Tennis? Golf? Hike? Tae-Bo? Yoga?

Advanced Exercise Routine: Home-Based—Dumbbells

Warm-up
Fifteen-minute run

- Squats
- Push-ups
- Dips
- Crunches
} Circuit 1

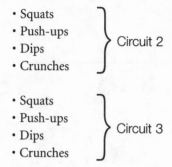

- Squats
- Push-ups
- Dips
- Crunches

} Circuit 2

- Squats
- Push-ups
- Dips
- Crunches

} Circuit 3

Three-minute run, jumping jacks, free dance, jump rope, or run up stairs

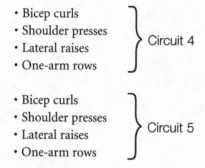

- Bicep curls
- Shoulder presses
- Lateral raises
- One-arm rows

} Circuit 4

- Bicep curls
- Shoulder presses
- Lateral raises
- One-arm rows

} Circuit 5

Three-minute run, jumping jacks, free dance, jump rope, or run up stairs

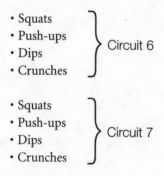

- Squats
- Push-ups
- Dips
- Crunches

} Circuit 6

- Squats
- Push-ups
- Dips
- Crunches

} Circuit 7

Fifteen-minute jog
Stretch and cool-down

Tuesday, Thursday

Forty-five-minute comfortable jog with periodic "power spurt" intervals of three minutes or longer

Saturday or Sunday (or both)

Something fun and active: tennis, golf, a hike, Tae-Bo, or yoga

Advanced Exercise Routine: Gym-Based

Warm-up
Fifteen-minute run

- Cable rows (or Lat pull-downs)
- Incline press machine
- Leg extensions
- Leg curls

} Circuit 1

- Cable rows (or Lat pull-downs)
- Incline press machine
- Leg extensions
- Leg curls

} Circuit 2

- Cable rows (or Lat pull-downs)
- Incline press machine
- Leg extensions
- Leg curls

} Circuit 3

Three-minute run on treadmill

- Bicep curls
- Shoulder presses
- Lateral raises

} Circuit 4

- Bicep curls
- Shoulder presses
- Lateral raises

} Circuit 5

Three-minute run on treadmill

- Leg press
- Push-ups
- Dips
- Crunches (or bicycles)

} Circuit 6

- Leg press
- Push-ups
- Dips
- Crunches (or bicycles)

} Circuit 7

Fifteen-minute jog
Stretch and cool-down

Tuesday, Thursday

Forty-five-minute comfortable jog with periodic "power spurt" intervals of three minutes or longer

Saturday or Sunday (or both)

Something fun and active. Tennis? Golf? Hike? Tae-Bo? Yoga?

Resources

Books on General Nutrition

Nutrition Made Simple, by Robert Crayhon, Ph.D. Probably the best general introduction to nutrition on the market from one of the most gifted teachers on the planet.

Nutritionally Incorrect, by Allan Spreen, M.D. An outstanding medical doctor who is also a superb nutritionist takes on the establishment.

Nutrition in a Nutshell, by Bonnie Minsky, M.A., C.N.S. Another wonderful introductory book for the general public.

Eating and Lifestyle Plans

Protein Power LifePlan, by Michael Eades, M.D., and Mary Dan Eades, M.D. If you haven't read their previous book, *Protein Power,* and you want to find out what they're about, this is the place to start, since it represents their most recent thinking. All sorts of interesting subjects are covered, including wonderful information on cholesterol. Be forewarned: Although brilliantly done, it is a bit dense for complete beginners, and goes into a lot of detail.

The Schwarzbein Principle, by Diana Schwarzbein, M.D. An excellent approach to lower carb living and the reasoning behind it from a top endocrinologist.

The Zone books, by Barry Sears, Ph.D. Take your pick, they're all good. For those who are not ready to give up fast food, *Seven Days in the Zone* tells you how to make those meals less damaging from a hormonal point of view.

The Living Beauty Detox Program, by Ann Louise Gittleman, M.S., C.N.S. Several plans for detoxifying your system and your environment written by one of the best nutritionists in America.

Eat Fat, Lose Weight, by Ann Louise Gittleman, M.S., C.N.S. More reasons why the low-fat mania is counterproductive, from the former director of the ultra-low-fat Pritikin Center.

The Balance, by Oz Garcia. Straight-shooting advice on how to eat right for your metabolic type.

Fit For Life: A New Beginning, by Harvey Diamond. Diamond's experience is inspiring and the book contains excellent information on detoxification.

Books on Vitamins and Supplements

The Nutraceutical Revolution, by Richard Firshein, D.O. Solid and accessible information on some of the superstars of nutritional therapy.

The Vita-Nutrient Solution, by Robert Atkins, M.D. I use this as a virtual text-book.

Immunotics, by Robert Rountree, M.D. One of America's best doctors shares strategies for boosting your bodys ability to defend itself against toxins.

Books on Psychology and Diet

Potatoes Not Prozac, by Kathleen Des Maisons, Ph.D. An excellent discussion of the brain chemistry of sugar addicts and how to use food to combat cravings.

The Crazy Makers, by Carol Simontacchi, M.S., C.C.N. A well-researched and compelling argument for the influence of modern processed food on behavior, especially relevant if you have children.

Books on Exercise

Fitness for Dummies, and *Weight Training for Dummies,* by Liz Neporent and Suzanne Schlosberg. There is simply nothing better on the market for beginners who want excellent and easy to understand advice about exercise.

Slow Burn, by Stu Mittleman. Solid and thoughtful advice on nutrition, exercise and life from a true original.

Books on Special Conditions and Situations

Diabetes: Prevention and Cure, by C. Leigh Broadhurst, Ph.D. I recommend this book for absolutely everybody—it is a storehouse of valuable information on nutrition, diet and the rationale for a lower carb approach.

Syndrome X, by Jack Challem, Burt Berkson, M.D., Ph.D., and Melissa Diane Smith. A very clear explanation of how insulin resistance works, why you don't want it and what to do about it.

Feast Without Yeast, by Bruce Semon, M.D., Ph.D., and Lori Kornblum. A good explanation for how diet can connect to a multitude of problems—includes a good cookbook.

Fight Fat After Forty, by Pamela Peeke, M.D., M.P.H. Brilliant explanation of the role of stress in weight gain.

The Liver Cleansing Diet, by Sandra Cabot, M.D. The importance of the liver in both health and weight maintenance, with some excellent and easy strategies for detoxification.

The False-Fat Diet, by Elson Haas, M.D. One of America's best nutritionally oriented medical doctors explains why many foods in your diet may be causing problems like bloating and weight retention, and what you can do about it.

The Memory Solution, by Julian Whitaker, M.D. An icon in the field of integrative medicine tells you how to keep your brain healthy and functioning throughout your life. Especially interesting to baby-boomers.

Cookbooks

Nourishing Traditions, by Sally Fallon. Subtitled *"The Guide to Politically Incorrect Nutrition,"* this book is nothing less than a must-have.

Generally Inspiring

Life Is an Attitude, by Dottie Billington, Ph.D. A lovely and inspiring little book about creating your life and rewriting your story.

Love for the Living, by Dan Saferstein, Ph.D. Very moving meditations on the meaning of marriage and life.

Hormone Management

Cenegenics Medical Institute
851 South Rampart Blvd., Suite 201
Las Vegas, NV 89128
1–888-YOUNGER

Hormones—testosterone, estrogen, DHEA, thyroid, and human growth hormone, to name a few—can and do have profound effects on mood, energy, vitality, weight, and aging. Presently, this is the best facility for providing state-of-the-art medical evaluation and treatment lans. It also works with many local doctors across the country.

Vitamins, Minerals, Supplements and the Like

Designs for Health Insitute (1–800–847–8302). I particularly like their Paleomeal (whey protein powder), but the whole product line is superb and affordable.

Metagenics (1–800–638–2848). Long a favorite of doctors, it also makes first-rate products.

Cenegenics Medical Institute (1–888-YOUNGER). If you like your vitamins and supplements in easy-to-take pre-packaged daily packs, these are the best formulas on the market.

Life Extension Institute (1–800–841–5433). This company makes wonderful, high-quality stuff, and also publishes a very well-done magazine called *Life Extension.*

Web Site

My site, **www.jonnybowden.com** will link you to other sites of interest, will keep you up-to-date on what I've been doing and will also link you to my radio show on eyada.com and my columns on ivillage.com and elsewhere. There are news items pertaining to health, nutrition and lifestyle, reviews of books and commentary on . . . well, just about everything.

INDEX